KNOW THYSELF

Your Body's Wisdom for
LIVING CONSCIOUSLY

Who you are and
how you function as an
integrated organ/gland energy system

Dean G. Allen, PhD

AH HA Publications

KNOW THYSELF:
Your Body's Wisdom for Living Consciously

ISBN: 978-0-9888012-0-2

Cover image by Shawn Hocking, shockingartwork.com
Back cover photo by Brenda Leap
Interior images by Radisha, Dianne Magel, and Bora Orcal

AH HA PUBLICATIONS
Boise, Idaho

Printed in the United States

Infrared science reveals how we unconsciously program our present functioning from our *past* trauma memory (of *emotional dysfunction*) to create our *present* physical diseases.

From this book, you can learn to see and be Who You Are energetically as twenty-three Spirit Life-force organ/gland energy systems and functions.

At the beginning and the end of every human problem, Life is a game of consciousness for control of our *decisions* in our moments of power. These *choices* are between our Spirit's Ways (of Love and Light that align with the Laws of energy) and the dragon's ways of deception, confusion and manipulation by using fear and force.

No matter the question
The answer's the same.
It's all about ENERGY.

It's Life's Only Game!

~ Dean G. Allen, PhD

Contents

Dedication

Dedicated to the Truth Seekers who seek their true Self!

This book is dedicated to raising human consciousness about who we are and how we function energetically to align with the Laws of Energy, and to continuing the research needed to develop an advanced, integrated science of Mind, Body and Spirit. This *integration* is the only thing that can provide a *real, Conscious Health Care Plan!*

This book has evolved over my many years of attempting to more clearly refine and clarify how life really works energetically, from my many years of studying psychology, observing clients, and personal interactions with other gifted professionals. But what I appreciate the most, I have learned from thousands of clients to whom I am *most* grateful for their strength and courage to take this *infrared* journey to *consciously and energetically 'connect their personal dots'* by observing their energy flow patterns.

Doing this with my clients since 1987 has for me profoundly clarified a much more refined view of energetic Reality about all humans. This book capitalizes the word 'Reality' because I am talking about energetic Reality or the Ways Reality exists as energy – described by Laws/Ways of energetic Reality (physics and metaphysics) at the most subtle and basic levels of *everything* because *everything is energy*!

This book is especially dedicated to those people who have made the most significant contributions to my life, beginning with my parents, Charlie and Elsie – both gifted, strong clear Spirits with pure hearts. (I didn't know how great I had it until I saw a much bigger picture later from other's in life.)

I also want to dedicate this book to my older brother Gene (C. Eugene Allen, Ph.D. in Food Science and Nutrition) for lighting my pathway to higher education (*our father's dream* was to be well educated, which he only fulfilled through us). Gene was the first in my family to find that uncharted pathway of education to get 'off the farm' and learn to know and find our passions that fulfill our divine purpose.

I am always inspired by *clear Spirits with pure hearts who follow their truth with pleasure* and I have worked with many other delightfully wise individuals like those mentioned here in my Acknowledgments who have had a most significant impact in my life.

Acknowledgments

I first met *Norm Shealy, MD, PhD,* in 1978 while doing my internship at the Boise State University Counseling Center, and was immediately inspired by his brilliant mind and courageous soul for doing everything he has done to advance health practices for victims of pain and degeneration. I only met Norm because he had made everyone so nervous at his first lecture on nutrition before lunch that they were afraid to eat with him! I had previously asked our director (who sponsored Dr. Shealy) if I could meet with Dr. Shealy when he was in Boise, and was first told that all of his time was booked up with senior Staff members. But after the lunch that followed Norm's presentation, I was asked if I would like to take Dr. Shealy to dinner. I said: "Absolutely!" I took him to the grocery store to get whatever he wanted and we cooked it on my grill at home. We had a great meal and great conversation! Thanks, Norm, for everything! (Norm's website is: http://www.norm-shealy.com/)

Then in 1987 I met *Joseph R. Scogna, Jr.,* whose personal serious and painful experiences directed him on a path that made him see energetic Reality clearly enough, long enough to be able to scientifically observe and connect how the human system *integrates* energetically between its *psychology, biology* and *physics.* Thank you, Joe, for your brilliant inductive mind that allowed you to so keenly observe Reality in such clear concepts that truly align with Who we humans already are organically and energetically!

Then in 1988 I met *Louise L. Hay* (of HayHouse Publishing), whose sharp, quick mind and gracious soul saw this work as being *"Light years ahead of any other form of therapy"* and tried to publish my first book, *Dancing with your Dragons,* but complications prevailed against that happening. I am most grateful to Louise for all she did for me in my early days. But most of all, thanks for the great times, the incredible meals (not to mention the fine wines), and the stimulating conversations we've shared from Los Angeles to Paris. (Louise's website is http://www.louisehay.com.)

And finally, in 2005, I met my loving, beautiful, wise and talented wife, *Kristy Knight Allen,* who is my late coming soul-mate and the love of my life! Thanks, Kristy, for just being who you are every day!

And I could never thank you enough for your significant editorial contributions to the many versions of this book that have been updated way too many times, already! Thanks, my love! My most recent significant connection is with *Dr. Mary Migliori (MD)* whom I first met as a client who soon connected the physical and emotional dots between her work and my work. We are now both starting (2013) to work together to integrate our work into an *integrative conscious health spa* practice.

Acknowledgements: To my long time best friends who have supported me over my life.

Charlie Poulsen was a student in my first "Psychology of Consciousness Course," which I taught in 1977, and we have remained close friends ever since even though it may seem that we have little in common!

I met *Fadia Nancy Rice* in Egypt in 1994 on a consciousness tour where I was a speaker. Knowing her Spirit has been one of the greatest joys of my life that began with a picture I took of her as we were each riding our camels across the desert, in Egypt, with the *three grand pyramids* in the background. Fadia is the one who taught me one of my favorite phrases that I use quite often: "God has a Plan."

I met *Aiko Aiyana* in Los Angeles in the mid 1990's and was always impressed with her keen mind and genteel character and came to also be impressed by the healer within that she has continued to develop over many years. We did some work together on the East Coast for a while when she became interested in the BodyTalker before she moved to Hawaii. We have very similar interests and plan to work together again soon.

I met *Caara Shayne* (an angel from the City of Angels – Los Angeles) in 2001. She shares many common interests with me in the areas of consciousness and media as well as being a major contributor to what it has taken to finally get this book published. We've shared many memorable times together in Venice Beach and Topanga, California, as well as camping with her and husband Scott.

(Her first video interview with me is on YouTube at *http://youtube.com/user/DGAllenPhD*. Her second is also on YouTube at: *http://www.youtube.com/watch?v=A76AWMKYci8&feature=youtu.be.*)

I met *Vicki Fisk* as a client in 2002 and within a week she made three dramatic changes in her life that she had pondered about for several years indecisively, until the resolution of her issues *suddenly* became clear after our first session! I found this very impressive. We still see each other often, whenever possible, to discuss anything and everything.

And last, but not least, to my *many other friends* (you know who you are) who have enriched my life immensely with our deep and rich connections.

I also dedicate this book to my *thousands of incredible clients* who came to me seeking clarity and were brave enough to face themselves so they could recognize *their own programming* and then do something about it.

Love and Light, and Many Thanks to All …
Dean G. Allen, PhD

Foreword

Personally Understanding Enlightened Functioning

By Kristy Knight Allen

If you have ever wondered if you were 'more than just a body' – this book is for you. It describes the entirety of Who You Are better than anything I've ever seen. It explains how our energy integrates perfectly, naturally and logically between our Spirit Self, our mental Self, our emotional Self as well as our physical Self in a way that is 'Self evident and undeniable.' This is because it uses concepts that are scientific and well documented from many years of research using infrared technology and *something inherent* in each of us that really does explain Who we are and how we function as human beings. And that *something inherent* is the language of the body itself! For me, this language puts it all together in such a way that leaves very little room for doubt about how the game of life really works energetically!

I feel so honored to recommend the man who wrote this book to you. I knew Dean for several years while we developed a friendship (we lived in separate towns and he always called me at midnight every night just to talk). Over time, this developed into a deep and abiding trust. One day I asked him, "What am I going to do with you? He was my best friend, but I could feel something else developing between us and yet marriage (after 2 tries) still seemed out of the question for me. After all, we were just friends, anyway. We talked about it and I'll never forget what Dean told me that day. He said, "Friendship based on trust is really all there is – and if you have that, nothing else matters. And if you *don't* have that, nothing else matters."

That was something to think about. And I did. After all, I always wanted to marry a man that was a true friend to my Spirit. Someone I could *trust*.

After several years and a lifetime of looking, it was revealed to me in a profound way that Dean was *the one for me*. It finally came to me how much I loved this *'nerd hot'* guy and how irreplaceable he was!

What a relief that a lifetime of looking was now over! Six months later, we got married and those who attended said that it was the best wedding they had ever witnessed. The ceremony ended as we both donned a pair of sunglasses – because I once asked Dean what our future was going to be like and he said, "It's going to be so bright – we're going to need sunglasses!"

And in spite of all life's challenges since then, he was right when he said: "When you do it the way it works, it works!"

After really getting to know him all these years, I respect his profound knowledge base – but even more, I respect his 'heart knowledge' that can see into the hidden places and can heal with compassion as well as the shine some enormous Light on this astounding science that he and the ones that came before him have discovered about what makes us all 'tick' energetically (which can now be tracked and measured using infrared science.)

According to the 'Order of the Magi' (an order of ancient knowledge) Dean is the "King of Knowledge." This King of Clubs is all about the accumulation and implementation of knowledge. But way beyond that, he also just happens to be the kindest and most caring soul I have ever met. And I can honestly say that I have gained *more* respect for him with each passing day in the 8 years I have known him.

The concept of feeling 'safe and worthy of love' was unknown to me before I met Dean Allen and suffice it to say how grateful I feel to now be able to call him my husband (after a courtship that put his beautiful Spirit to the test entirely until my walls came down and I felt safe enough to be more real in the ways I related to him.) When you have never felt safe in that way before (to be the real 'you' in a relationship), it's a game changer. I can also say with certainty that it is a direct result of the Language of the Body being implemented in my life that led to recognizing who Dean was (when, in a moment of clarity, I was able to peer into times past and know without a doubt that I knew him 'before.')

I feel that a lot of credit goes to our previous relationships we soul contracted into so we could learn the great lessons of contrast. I was used to being in relationships that got *worse over time* as respect and trust was lessened with a toxic emotional build up going on with both parties – because *neither of us knew how to play the game in a rejuvenative fashion* in order to create a strong and Spirit filled relationship.

What I have since learned is that sometimes we cannot appreciate true connection until we have tortured ourselves by disconnected relationships. After all, it was these hard fought for lessons that gave Dean and I the wisdom to cradle, nurture and evolve our relationship into what we have now. There is so much to be said for being with someone that *feels like home* to you after feeling estranged in every primary relationship you have ever had before that. That's the power of trust in love. For those who have found it, true love is less about luck and more about that kind of trust that makes all Spirits feel 'at home.'

However, in order to have recognized this harmony, a marriage within ourselves had to have already occurred before we met. Because how can we recognize an energy that is foreign to us? To be honest, I almost missed this harmony in my life. Harmony is the great lesson of the heart organ – that teaches us to tune in to and recognize it when we feel and see it – so we can trust it and embrace it instead of running the other way because it is so different that we 'don't know what to do with it' when it's standing right there in front of us (which is what I almost did). And without an insatiable thirst for something real and an inner search for harmony for almost 50 years, I might not have recognized what harmony could feel like in my relationship with Dean.

But I had a lot more than heart issues (which I found out according to my first scan). My journey of healing before I met Dean led me toward many different modalities, but all left me with the same kidney issue that I had suffered from for over 20 years (as well as many other maladies both physical and emotional). The interesting thing is that my mother died from kidney issues, so finding out from Dean that this issue was about discerning and discriminating the toxic emotional situations in my life was more than interesting since made so much sense to me because it was an exact fit and precisely described my life up to that point!

My point to all this is that knowledge is power and putting that knowledge to use in our relationships is what this book is all about. (This why I believe Dean's work really shines.)

By paying closer attention to our Spirit messages *within us,* and by understanding their meanings and implementing them, we become more unified with our Spirit, and duality begins to wane within us. This has a direct result in our relationships. This 'oneness mentality' automatically changes our outer world as well. (It is how the 'as above, so below' idea becomes implemented in a conscious fashion.)

This books shows us with a remarkable clarity how we can turn our weaknesses into our strengths. It shows us how to shine the light of energetic Reality into the dark places of our lives so that we are no longer confused as to *how we got to where we are*. And more than that, it can show us exactly how to *get to where we want to go* if we apply these principles and Laws toward becoming more consciously directed by Spirit Life-force energy.

Dean once told me that he attracts *clients who have strong Spirits* that are in charge of their life. When I asked how that happens, he said it boils down to Spirits who are capable of seeking truth with pleasure, (the requirement and signature of any Spirit Being). Each of us can achieve a quantum level leap in consciousness when we are able to seek truth with pleasure and implement that alignment into our lives. This is especially true when we align with the energetic Truth (the light of truth that is based on the Spiritual and natural Laws of energy).

The key is to have a strong enough Spirit to recognize truth when we see it! And, even if it is different than what we were *taught* or *thought* it was – to still have the courage to see and follow it any-way – because we are heart prompted to know that it is the inner truth of all humans because it is the energetic Truth! Following these ener-getic Laws is what I call going from the *outside church* – to the *inside church*. Because no matter what our affiliations are, it's the direction all Spirits are going, anyway. And it is also what will eventually bring us all together into a much more peaceful world.

Energy follows energy which is why *like attracts like*. I love meet-ing people who have done enough personal work to be interested in consciousness issues, which is why I have always enjoyed meeting any of Dean's clients that have been attracted to this work. Because of their desire to seek truth with pleasure, they are all in a class by themselves!

It takes an enormous amount of courage to not only *seek the truth* – but when you are blessed enough to find it, to also be disciplined enough to *implement* it into your life. But once you do, you will grow in ways never thought possible to you before. Our basic power *that is our birthright* has literally and always been within us – in each organ and gland in our bodies (though this fact has had to be rediscovered through countless ages). This is why we have always had the power to change our world into something that works according to the Spiritual and natural Laws of energy. And when we do this, we can also dramati-cally lengthen our lives, as well as strengthen the way we live them.

Now, accessing these natural powers within us won't be so hard when the language of the organs and glands in the body becomes more available through practitioners that have access to The BodyTalker technology. It uses infrared for a scientific energy reading, coupled with the body's own built in a read out and interpretation of the energetic signature of each organ/gland's energy flow.

This language becomes a mirror that shows how your power on the 253 circuits of your body is flowing (creating regeneration), or blocked (creating degeneration) as it accurately interprets (to a thousandth of a degree) exactly what your body has been saying to you in the way of encoded messages. These messages may look like diseases, disorders or dysfunctions (or a life that is happy and filled with the fulfillment of our divine intent). But the question is always: "Are we getting the message?" Getting these messages is what this book is all about.

Healers and mystics on the planet at this time are pioneers on the frontiers of consciousness! I have had a unique position as one of the editors of this book to live with one of those pioneers. Also, I have had a unique opportunity to be able to not only live with the wisdom in this book, but the amazing man who wrote it! Working on this book for several years has allowed me to see myself in a way I never before thought possible. And what a pleasure it has been for me to become acquainted with the divine secrets of the Language of the Body!

Dean has distilled so many lifetimes of experiential knowledge into this book about the ways we are designed to work, so life doesn't need to be a mystery to us any longer as our divine intent (what we came here to do) sneaks up to greet us (once our energy blocks are dealt with and our circuits are clear)!

This energetic signature for each of us has always been locked up in our organs and glands. They are the 'Rosetta Stone' for how each of us works energetically as 253 circuits of potential Spirit Life-force energies flowing through us as The Light of each organ's truth.

We can now consciously understand these secrets so we can process our life at the *speed of light* by understanding the personal language of each organ/gland energy system. Our original design allows us to see how we are meant to *integrate* our Life-force energy on all four levels of ourselves: Spiritually, mentally, emotionally as well as physically.

Our visible spectrum is only 1/88th of our reality, and yet as a species, we still pay most of our attention to our physical realm. And in doing this, it becomes more difficult to see the obvious, though at first, more subtle energetic Reality clearly. But this must happen in order to turn things around after seeing how our more subtle aspects of emotional functioning are designed to integrate with our spiritual and mental as well as the physical levels of energy.

Dean is always saying: "The *human system is not designed to degenerate and die.*" I mean, "Who talks like that?" But after seeing how this game works in my own life, I can see that as long as we are controlled by our 'drag,' we don't know what we are doing energetically *enough* to make our lives really *work* so we can regenerate and rejuvenate. But if we can learn to once again consciously flow with our Life-force energy spontaneously (the way we are designed to regenerate and rejuvenate), perhaps old expectations around disease and death won't have to be our inevitable conclusion as we become more conscious of new and never before thought of options as they become more available.

As you study this book and find out what this 'drag' on our Spirit Life-force (what we affectionately call our 'dragon') looks like, sounds like, and feels like in each organ and gland – you will be better able to see what is going on in your own life, because these energies affect everyone that is human with 253 circuits the same way. This is the insight that we already know on a very deep level – and therefore, it is not too hard to grasp (though Dean has always said that he can teach children this language easier than adults because of how they have been set in their ways).

However, the language itself takes time to 'grock.' The gist of it is that dragons have short term solutions – with long term problems; and Spirits are challenged with short term problems that provide long term solutions. The good news is – that any Great Spirit solution involves potentially short term challenges (like learning *your organ/gland language,* for instance), but the end result will always have a long term solution in mind.

The dragon is just another word for unconsciousness. Determining whether the drag on Spirit Life-force has been running our decision making process is what this book is all about. Before this great knowledge has been incorporated into our consciousness, it may be difficult to understand how much this may be happening to us, but finding out is well worth the effort. Implementing this language can take years of discipline and just plain hard work. It takes a certain amount of time to not only uncover the unconscious dragons that have been making our lives so difficult, but to figure out *why these actions were directed by philosophies that could never work (except to degenerate) energetically over time.*

The good news about this undisciplined dragon is that it can become disciplined by the light of energetic Reality. And instead of making up scenarios out of our worst fears, we can consciously get ahead of those fears and use the dragon's innate talents of survival and protection ONLY when we actually need to be protected vs. the 'trauma dramas' that the undisciplined dragon likes to keep us in while we are still in the dark about what is causing these 'drags' on each of our circuits.

I recently heard the statement: *"The distance between our dreams and reality equals action."* After 8 years, I am just beginning to understand this as I get that it is much, much more than just seeing. Because all points for getting what you want in life are given to us for not only seeing, but *doing!*

Infrared teaches us so much about what we don't yet know and that is because it covers not only what we see, but what we don't see. And the visible spectrum is only a tiny part of our entire energetic Reality – so learning to know what we cannot see and understanding how it works energetically, is of critical importance to how consciously we live our lives! The way that fits into what I am saying can be best summed up by this statement from the book *"Steering by Starlight"* by Martha Beck: "External circumstances do not create feeling states. Feeling states create external circumstances." In other words, energy forms the physical, not the other way around – which is what makes our thoughts and emotions so important to pay attention to.

I have now concluded with certainty based on my personal observations that the subtle aspects of Who we are energetically – are indeed the most important in regard to what we are creating in our lives Spiritually, mentally, emotionally as well our physical body. This is because Spirit Life-force energy is mentally programmed into emotional feelings that manifest in our bodies with messages about how life works and doesn't work!

This means that the physical body is the final dumping ground of energy. This appears to be the major problem in our healthcare system, because the physical body still is the most obvious and often the first place people look to for the answers to individual dysfunctions. And for the most part, the etheric causes for these diseases are largely *unknown in the realm of our present day 'health care.'*

Who knew that the body held these answers in an obvious language in the organs and glands this whole time? And that the energetic light that shines in the wisdom of these organs and glands (if consciously enacted for what they are designed to do) could fix every single problem that we face?

As human beings, we are made up of 253 circuits of personal powers that are designed to spontaneously flow with Spirit Life-force energy. But most of us really don't have a clue how to consciously do this because this profound information has not yet become largely known. However, once we know this language, we are much better equipped with the ability to make the kinds of regenerative decisions that keep Spirit Life-force flowing in us. This is the power of this book!

I see this book changing everything to do with the healing fields conceptually as we begin to look scientifically at where and how and why the dysfunctional energy begins spinning south in the etheric fields (spiritual, mental and emotional bodies) long before it ever manifests in the physical realm. These concepts allow us to see *ahead of the curve clearer and quicker* (a phrase used often in this book because it is the goal for using the language) to figure out how to turn our energy around before we dysfunction, degenerate, become diseased and headed for death on the physical level.

Dean is the only person I know with enough hindsight and foresight to write a book called **"Know ThySelf,** *your Body's Wisdom for Living Consciously"* about how the mind-body system truly works energetically as an *integrated* system that includes our 4 bodies (Spiritual, mental, emotional and physical). His entire personal as well as professional lifetime has led up to the sharing of this very important work. Someone finally put the pieces together about who we are and how we function energetically as a Spirit Life-force energy system – and was able to do the clinical research with clients over a sufficient amount of time to scientifically *back it up!*

Finally, we have some hard scientific evidence about Who we really Are (vs. some of the 'woo woo' New Age stuff that comes out with no real measurable evidence). Once you see it, the body's own language that is built right in to every human is *undeniable*. And now this language including an accurate measuring tool that uses infrared (The BodyTalker), allows us to see *beyond the rainbow* and shows us what is 'Self Evident' about Who we Are and how we function as human beings.

But Dean did not figure this science out on his own. And, he has always given full credit to the many scientists and great minds that came before him, especially to the works of Elmer Green and the brilliant Joseph Scogna (who died at the tender age of thirty-nine). Dean was a researcher in Biofeedback right after Elmer Green's work was initiated regarding the mind/body connection (when the Menninger Clinic was doing research on migraine headaches). Before that, there was a glaring lack of scientific research involving the mind body connection, so Dean has seen a lot of theories come and go since he has been in on the evolvement of this specific *mind-body science* from the beginning.

But if it wasn't for Joseph Scogna, Dean would have had a lot less information to go on as far as putting the whole picture together – so Joe gets a huge standing ovation for what he found out about Who we Really Are energetically as organ/gland systems that work as an integrated Whole in every human. Scogna had only a high school education and yet he made an enormous contribution to us all through his astounding discoveries surrounding this body of work! (Dean will tell you about his personal involvement with Joe in his own story.)

To me, it has been like that track and field event where the runners pass the baton to their team members. They each build on the legacy that went before them as they push further and further toward the collective consciousness finish line in their field. It took many lifetimes to discover and re-discover the knowledge presented in this book. *It then took someone to spend his entire professional life testing it as a clinician and researcher*. But it hasn't been easy being a pioneer in his field of work. Since Dean was not plugged into the health care 'status quo' system with insurance, etc., Dean's work has largely consisted of a clientele that for the most part had to seek him out from word of mouth referrals. And in the beginning there were times when things were lean as well as times when he found himself the anti-aging specialist for the stars in Hollywood (those clients who had no problem affording Dean's very valuable time)! But Dean is first and foremost a scientist (PhD in Clinical Psychology). And I commend his uncanny ability to see into all of Who we Are energetically – using not only his incredible insight and wisdom, but by using The BodyTalker technology that reflects a mirror image of the specific encoded energetic messages every organ/gland energy system of our body reveals in a brilliantly cohesive way!

Louise Hay (HayHouse Publishing) was his first client and said that Dean's work is "...*light years ahead of any other form of therapy*" and I concur. The work becomes a constant internal practice once you learn the language. After doing the work for eight years myself, it has become *much easier* to recognize, in the moment, the unconscious places that I operate from. This is a familiar comment from Dean's client base because when we understand and tune in to the more subtle aspects of our Selves, we can't help becoming more able to figure out 'how, when, where and why' we keep repeating patterns that do not work.

With the infrared BodyTalker science, we can always stay aware of where our actual Spirit Life-force blockages are. The Language of the Body then tells us how to decode this information into the unconscious decisions we are making that are creating our problems. It's powerful stuff because it is about how we are designed to work, using our very own organ/gland Language that works on all four levels, so we can see the grand design of our lives past just the physical level.

My work with Dean literally saved my life. And like I said before, since my mother died of kidney disease – it was looking like that was the direction I was headed as well – until I turned my kidney energy around after eight months of strenuous personal re-evaluation and work. I had to discipline my dragon – (in this case, my kidney dragon) as I figured out how to filter the toxic emotional situations out of my life (as indicated by my kidney symptoms) instead of continuing to endure them.

In spite of seeing many MD's, no doctor ever told me anything about my *kidney emotional function* until I ran into this infrared science. Also, my liver emotional functioning went from the unconscious liver dysfunction (of emotionally staying hopeless and disappointed), to being hopeful and having a dream to focus on by rekindling my 20 year singing career and getting my new *Spiritual, transformative songs* out to the world.

Before I discovered this astounding work, my dragon energy lived in the 'cave' of my unconsciousness and was running my life (since I was already showing physical effects on almost all of my organs and glands). In my professional life as a healer, I had begun to figure out my way in the energy world which had always profoundly interested me. So, after I set aside my singing career for a time, I became a Reiki Master, delved into the fascinating world of NLP, became a Master level Rapid Eye Technician (and had also previously worked for a chiropractor doing homeopathic research). *But nothing could have prepared me for the mind-blowing aspects of the Human Divine Design that Dr. Allen presented to me on my first session!* It was my exact Spiritual, mental, and emotional blueprint that was manifesting itself in my physical world! And the exciting part was – that I could now finally understand it as it became decoded in a way that was perfectly understandable.

I had always wanted to understand what my body was saying to me, and I got my wish that day (along with the many years of doing this work that have followed)! My first dose of Dean's insight, delivered with country humor (like Dr. Phil on steroids) allowed me to literally see how each organ/gland actually works energetically on an infrared readout that over time could track and measure my progress.

As a Rapid Eye technician, I knew that sleep is a natural way to process massive amounts of information. And after laughing and crying intensely during that first session as well as afterward, I slept for almost three days just processing the enormous work I had done on myself! Dean says that this is not an uncommon response to one's first session because of the amount of *new information* being processed.

I usually don't like to use the words, *wrong* or *right*, but until I found this science, I didn't really know one way or another exactly what an 'energetically correct decision' was! But once I saw clearly how the game worked, I found I had done things energetically *'wrong'* my whole life while thinking I was doing them energetically *'right.'* In other words, I thought I was rejuvenating when I was really degenerating!

I now know it was all about the ways I had not discerned and discriminated among the energies and people in my life before. Instead, I had spent most of my energy *trying to figure out how to make things work that could never work!* No wonder I was being drained of my energy! I thought this was being *Spiritual, nice and longsuffering* (as if 'suffering long' was a good thing). But when I figured it out, I could actually see the foolish price I had paid to try to *do it the way it couldn't work,* because of how costly it was to my organ/gland systems energetically in the long run.

After this first session, I asked myself, "Why was this not taught to me as a child in grade school?" I felt robbed and cheated, as if I had been making the recipe for life without all the ingredients all my life! That was when I realized what a pioneer Dean really is (as well as all those who went before to contribute to this work).

The clinical research that Dean has done since 1987 needed to be done to scientifically validate Joe Scogna's re-discoveries about the emotional functions of the organs and glands (Joe always said his work was a "*re*-discovery of our long lost blueprints") which is why he never said he *created* them.

It is clear to me that this profound insight was always the basis of spiritual work in each and every religion before the true religions became corrupted. After that, we saw symbolisms around 'temples' that were really always talking about *the temple that houses our Spirit* – which has always been **our bodies! After all, our organ/gland circuitry was designed to plug in to Spirit Life-force messages on a continual basis!** Missing this key piece of information could have clarified so much for us instead of the inestimable price tag of human suffering that the lack of knowing this inherent language has created!

After Dean became acquainted with the basics of this idea, Dean needed to see firsthand how it all fits into an integrated system. Then there was the challenge to see to it that this design could be properly read (as well as interpreted) in the same exact impeccable language that only our Source Creator could have imagined with such precision and Divine Intellect! It was hard to believe it at first, but now here he is twenty-five years later using our *body as evidence* of Who We Are and How We function with infrared science. And the exciting part is the long term implications of this that we are only just now tapping into.

The *organ/gland language* isn't just any language. It is the language of how humans process their emotions so we can spin our energy north toward rejuvenation versus spinning it south toward degeneration (which led to one of my favorite Dean quotables like, *"You can't go north when you're going south,"* (my personal favorite), and *"The primary human problem is confusion."*

The way I see it, a person would have to get clear enough to even begin to be able to put so many pieces together from so many places – so that person could resurrect this integrated knowledge – and clearly, that has been Dean's challenge along with so many others who have contributed to this 'body' of work.

So, this may seem like it is new on the planet (but there is no doubt in my mind that our beloved ancient brothers and sisters from more advanced civilizations knew these secrets as well, which is the reason they lived such long lives). It is an incredible Light – and an amazing and graceful evidence of Who We Really Are *As The Light!*

Our present and future joy as humans is all about this unveiling party around Who We Really Are. Arthur Schopenhauer said, "All truth passes through three stages. First, it is *ridiculed*. Second, it is *violently opposed*. Third, it is *accepted as being self-evident*."

This language of the body is Self-evident truth…literally! It is convincing and undeniable because it is our most basic design and is the way all humans function energetically. Every symptom is a message that can be tracked, decoded and acted upon. The question is: "Are we following Spirit Life-force energy promptings, or not?"

By learning to use our body's language, we will more easily be able to relate to each other as Spiritual Beings in a human body as we pioneer our way to clearly see and master the subtle aspects of our Being. Because of the many scientific correlations from Joe Scogna, Elmer Green, Dean Allen and a host of others whose research led up to it, the wisdom of our body has now been scientifically decoded, understood, and clinically validated so we can now implement these insights into our daily lives.

A wise man once said the following:

"The man who is enslaved by his passions or worldly prejudices cannot be initiated into wisdom; he must reform or he will never attain. Meanwhile, he cannot be an adept, for wisdom signifies a person who has achieved by will and by work. The man who loves his own opinions and fears to part with them, who suspects new truths, who is unprepared to doubt everything rather than admit anything on chance, should close this book: for him it is *useless and dangerous*. He will fail to understand it, and it will trouble him (while if he should find divine the meaning, there will be a still greater source of disquietude). If you hold by anything in the world more than by reason, truth and justice; if your will be uncertain and vacillating, either in good or evil. If logic alarm you, or the naked truth make you blush; if you are hurt when accepted errors are assailed; condemn this work straight away. Do not read it; let it cease to exist for you; but at the same time do not cry it down as dangerous. The secrets which it records will be understood by an elect few and will be reserved by those who understand them." ~ *Eliphas Levi, 1896*

I would like to see this book get out into the world – not to just an 'elect few' but to all those who want to feel the literal power of their implementation of Who they really are as Spirit Beings! "**Know Thy-Self,** *your Body's Wisdom for Living Consciously*" is best used to help people realize the fact that they are truly Spirits with the ability to tap into all energetic powers provided to them from Source Energy on all of their circuits! And when we do this – we are literally unlimited in our possibilities as Beings of Light.

Deepak Chopra wrote, *"Every time you are tempted to react in the same old way, ask if you want to become a prisoner of your past – or a pioneer of your future."*

That's what this book is all about. It's very content is pioneering. It assists each of us in recognizing what Dean has always said: "Consciousness is the only elegant solution to human problems." This is because consciousness is the only way we can break from our old reactive ways and transform them into a future that manifests what Dean calls our divine intent.

Spirit energy makes decisions with the future in mind; but the undisciplined dragon (the 'drag' on Spirit Life-force energy) doesn't have the foresight to see how present decisions affect the future (which is why our undisciplined dragon decisions are mainly concerned about survival in the moment). Understanding the differences in these two energies that the 'yin/yang' symbol is made up of (representing the 'whole' of each of us) is the key to everything in regard to successful, regenerative decisions that can really make a difference in our lives *long term.*

Now, these long term solutions can be made with confidence in the form of actions that our Spirit has always wanted to make (but didn't have the power when ruled by the short term consciousness of the undisciplined 'drag' on Spirit Life-force energy). And instead of being at odds with this energy inside of us, we can truly appreciate the dragon for its gifts and then discipline it with the light of energetic Reality so it can evolve from being in the *cave of unconsciousness* to the *lake of emotional healing,* to the *sky of soaring personal power* as this disciplined dragon's divine intent becomes our greatest support in the times of survival when our Spirit needs it the most.

This is why this highly disciplined 'dragon in the sky' is the 5,000 year old mythical dragon that the Chinese celebrate even today! With the Language of the Body finally being re-discovered and implemented – we can learn to make the kinds of well-honed decisions and actions (according to the Spiritual and natural Laws of energy) that will work energetically toward a more unified consciousness from within us as well as from without (because one 'Reality' seems to be a reflection of the other).

Then, as we see more clearly how the game works, we can make decisions that can unify how we play it in our governments, health systems, and everything that relates to us energetically. This language can better enable us to become vessels of Spirit in all of our 253 circuits as we begin to uncover and use our gifts and talents to Be All that we were Source Designed to Be.

In fact, there is no doubt in my mind that the implementation of this knowledge can eventually create the ***end of duality within us.*** Because, while all Spirits may not agree on everything – if we can begin to use the 'straight and narrow path' of energy as our guide, can you imagine what a different world we can create together? And this is what gives me the hope that we will all soon graduate from a world of ***survival*** into the Golden Age of ***Thrive-All!***

Kristy Knight Allen,

9/9/2013

KNOW THYSELF

Preface

How Infrared Science Tracks and Decodes Electrical Flow

Know Thyself summarizes twenty-five years of my scientific insights and discoveries gleaned from observing and tracking thousands of client's *energy flow patterns* to decode their unconscious (triggered reactive trauma memory) decisions programming their Life-force energy into *dysfunctions* in their body's health, their business functions and relationship problems.

This book is called *Know Thyself* because it explains how the body's different energetic levels of density function together as an *integrated* whole. It provides a whole new level of clarity for how organ/gland energies perform our personal integrated functioning. The new/old Language of the Body upgrades our consciousness about our Self – from old limiting ideas to new more complete energetic realities – that can allow us to process our life more clearly and quickly.

The material in this book is for the purpose of shining light on new and more conscious directions that will evolve us into new dimensions of twenty-first century consciousness. We can anticipate continuous accelerating changes in our world, which will force us to accelerate our clarity in order to even be able to process our lives in a more coherent manner to manifest our divine intent.

Scientifically tracking personal energy flow patterns allows us to become more consciously connected to our most basic powers and messages relating to our *physical* symptoms, *emotional* dysfunctions and *mental* confusions, so we can create our *solutions*.

Becoming conscious of our organ/gland energy messages enlighten us about who we are and how we function at our most basic level of energetic functioning. This is essential to give us the power to create our solutions.

Seeing and knowing who we are and how we function energetically allows us to consciously use our twenty-three organ/gland energy tools to play by the Rules to win our Game of Life. Becoming consciously aligned with the force of the Rules, Laws and Ways of energy defines how we win more points and have fewer penalties with decisions that express our truth more clearly, quickly and appropriately.

> *What I have learned is that 'REALITY'*
> *Is not what most people think it to be!*

If we think and act according to *unreal ideas* about 'Reality' (Laws/ Ways of energy), then *confusion* becomes our primary human problem! (If you doubt confusion *is* our primary human problem, then just watch the evening news!)

When Reality's energetic truth is not understood with sufficient concepts to provide conscious clarity, sub-optimal confused thinking only 'kind of,' 'sort of' reflects true energetic Reality. That's because confused *concepts* do not fuse with energetic Reality (the Reality of how our unconscious subtle energy (without drag) flows/aligns with the Laws of energy to *regenerate* our Spirit Life-force).

In car racing, if we were to 'show up' as being *confused about our vehicle,* we would be told immediately that we *do not qualify* to drive our vehicle on the *track* because of the high probability of danger to our Self and others! This is true only because of our *confusion* about operating our vehicle through our *life*! We would be a danger to ourselves and others from being unqualified to drive with sufficient *performance* to ensure *safety* first then *fulfillment* for all!

If we are living in a body on planet earth, then we all have to play the game of life. It's apparently what we signed up for. The rules are the laws and ways of energy. And the tools are our twenty three organ/ gland energies. However, if we are confused about the rules and tools of the game, then where does this leave us if living our life just so happens to be totally dependent upon how life's game works energetically? In other words, if we are confused about the Rules and Tools needed to play our game of life, we can't even get started!

The first step to solving confusion is getting *clarity and consciousness* for how we achieve and maintain homeostasis (either by 'drag' or 'expression') through our Spirit Life-force energy flow. Then, our next step is to be sufficiently *conscious, in the moment,* to perceive and make use of our organ/gland energy *tools* so we perform in alignment with the Ways of the *Rules* that align with our *Spirit's Love and Light*.

What we humans are most confused about is who we are and how we function energetically. This confusion greatly diminishes our ability to see how we need to perform to regenerate and rejuvenate our Spirit Life-force energy in order to claim our personal power and direct our lives, personally, professionally and socially.

Infrared tracking of our electrical energy flow (electrons) between all of our organs and glands provides scientific clarify about our confusions over how our twenty-three organ/gland energy systems function to either *regenerate* or *degenerate*. These twenty-three systems determine 100% of who we are! They show how our Life-force energy flows as an *integration* of physical effects (symptoms/messages), from emotional dysfunctions and their mental/memory/consciousness that programs our Spirit Life-force energy to flow/drag, which either regenerates or degenerates. Infrared scanning does this by tracking our electrical energy flow patterns between our twenty-three organ/gland energy systems of 253 two-way (binomial) circuits of power.

The organ/gland language uses our inherent organ/gland energy functions' order of degeneration (revealed from radiation studies) to decode our blockage patterns, as we become conscious of how and what unconscious decisions are creating our problems! And once we do that, we finally have conscious choices (and without too much drag we'll make the regenerative decision)!

The organs and glands are recording devices that act like subtle emotional energy receptors. When we make unconscious/conscious decisions that either degenerate our Spirit Life-force energy, *or* regenerate our Life-force, each organ/gland records this energy experience in memory.

I have used this *organically formatted infrared science* of organ/gland electrical energy flow with every client since 1987, to decode their personal programming. This allows me to see my clients' energetic world more like how they experience it. This helps me help them enlighten the *'drag' on their Life-force* (what we refer to as the 'dragon') that shadows and obscures their Spirit's power and prevents them from perceiving and expressing their truth.

Over time, clients become more conscious so they can perceive more clearly and quickly, so they can take more appropriate, decisive

actions that are effective and productive. They can then express their personal truth more effectively to claim their personal power, which regenerates their health.

Clarity is the powerful tool that allows us to play our Game of Life the Way it was designed to work energetically. This is how we get more 'points' from clear, quick decisions that direct effective actions, which give us our personal power in the moment.

This is our challenge in our Life's Energy Game! It faces every human, every day, in every way, in every aspect of our lives!

The consciousness about our choices, decisions and actions determines our alignment with the 'force' of the 'Laws of energy.' Clearly aligned choices and actions give us our *personal power,* just like the gymnast who *integrates* what she *sees* and *feels* into a clear plan to *perform* by aligning her body with the force of the Laws of energy. When she does this, her body flows with that 'positive energetic force' (from the Laws of energy being congruently followed) in such a Way that her performance aligns with the grace and beauty that earns her a Gold Medal!

Life works the same way with everything. Every person's life is challenged by these same Laws of energy every day. This is because the *subtle aspects of reality* are the prime unconscious causes that determine the effects or outcomes in our lives. For this reason, it is very important for each of us to know how our God-given organ/gland tools are designed to play our Game of Life so we may consciously choose to *regenerate,* and choose to not *degenerate* our energy (in our moments of power).

This book provides all seekers of personal truth with a view further down the path and 'ahead of the curve' to show how our personal tools provide insightful, natural strategies for processing our lives so we all can live more consciously.

CONSCIOUSNESS SYSTEMS is the name of my company, along with my Conscious Living Project being developed at our **Hot Springs Retreat** in southern Idaho.

My success in using the infrared organ/gland energy system has resulted in many delighted clients whose testimonials you can read by going to the client feedback section that I have on my website: http://

DGAllenPhD.com. This website will continue to provide more things from new sciences to help shine light on our human pathway to personal enlightenment as this project evolves.

....

Author's note: I have intentionally capitalized the words *Laws, Rules, Spirit* and *Ways,* and in some instances, *Reality, Love, Light, Tools* and *Who,* to distinguish them as all being the "bigger Reality" (energetic Reality) of Spirit Ways, Laws and Rules of *energy* that are outside of any individual "little r" reality. Since this differentiation is a major premise of this book, I feel this style is important to help the reader clearly comprehend this energetic perspective.

KNOW THYSELF

Introduction

Understanding Enlightened Functioning

I have come to realize that *confusion is the primary cause of all human problems.* The reason this is true is that when we make our decisions based on concepts that do not 'fuse' with energetic Reality, this confusion creates a cycle of dysfunction, fear and trauma that defensively drains our resources and imprisons our Spirit. This base problem stems from a lack of clarity for who we truly are as Spirit Life-force energies living in a physical body, designed to function *consciously* to regenerate and fulfill our divine intent, *or* to function *unconsciously* from past memory to degenerate from confused actions.

The only effective solution to this dilemma is first to see more clearly who we are energetically. This allows us to understand and practice performing how we are designed to function and regenerate so we are more readily choosing conscious choices that align with the natural Laws of physics and the metaphysical Ways of subtle Spirit Life-force energy.

This book is the culmination of my many years of research and clinical work in this exciting new field of human potential based on some unique insights from what is called: "The organ/gland degenerative order," revealed from the human radiation studies from Nagasaki, Hiroshima and Three-Mile Island. This was re-discovered by the late Joseph R. Scogna, Jr. when in the early 1970's he began *connecting the dots between natural organ/gland thoughts, feelings and functions.*

Many of the organ/gland descriptive words used by Scogna to describe our natural organ/gland emotional feeling functions are the same words I use in this book to describe these natural organ/gland feelings. I do this because only those words precisely describe and define those organ/gland emotional experiences that are naturally associated with specific organ/gland emotional energies.

The scientific tool I use to track/decode human energy flow patterns is called **'The BodyTalker,'** which is an *emotional infrared scanner.* I

23

have used infrared science with clients since 1994 [see client feedback at http://dgallenphd.com/13743.html]. It provides an unprecedented level of insight into our programmed *integrated* functions of human power, behavior and disease. This technology mirrors an 'organic' (another useful meaning for organic) format that reveals how our human physical, emotional and mental systems are *mirror images of each other*. This insight reveals how the human body, mind and Spirit energies integrate to work together to create health, or work against each other to *disintegrate*, degenerate and *create disease and illness*.

By tapping into the stored memory of traumas that subconsciously control and direct our life and body, we are shown not only how we are programmed, but also how we can untangle and reprogram ourselves in order to live healthier, happier lives in a more fulfilling, productive and purposeful way.

How Infrared Science Tracks and Decodes Our Electrical Energy Flow

The discovery of this remarkable system dates back to the radiation studies done on the victims of H-bomb and power plant radiation. These studies reveal that the human body's twenty-three organ/gland energy systems degenerate in a very specific and particular order in every case when exposed to such radiation. Such intense radiation *accelerates the aging process* so one 'ages' in minutes and hours as much as what would normally take years and decades.

This *degenerative order* of organ/gland Spirit Life-force energy reveals an *'organ gland language'* of who we are and how we function energetically as an 'integrated constant' which is true for every human in terms of format and different for every human in terms of their specific history and programming.

This is the starting point for identifying our own individual differences. This new approach gives us a unique, new way to understand ourselves, using what I have termed *'organic psychology'* – that is a hybrid of *psychology* (mind), *biology* (body) and *physics* (Spirit Life-force) I call *'Psycho-Bio-Physics.'*

In 1974 I began my doctoral work at Utah State University that led to my Clinical Psychology dissertation research using biofeedback to try to scientifically connect human mind, body and Spirit Life-force energy functions. The overall objective of my research was to make specific scientific connections for how our mind connects to (as well as functions and communicates with) our body.

In 1982 I completed my research and then worked in the corporate world as a *wellness consultant* doing stress management. I used biofeedback to train personnel and executives about what their stress was, and how to *avoid* it and better *process* it. However, I quickly became frustrated practicing psychology *without any scientific tools to integrate more complete wellness solutions.* As a result, in 1987 I abandoned my psychology practice because it was very depressing for me. The reason for this was that I did *not* have the tools I needed to give my clients what they were coming to me to get (which to me would be a clear understanding of who they are and how they function so they could better process their life clearer, quicker and more productively).

Six months later, in 1987, I met Joseph Scogna (now deceased) and learned about his discoveries. I recognized immediately that he had *discovered how to use infrared science to reveal the subtle-energy connections* I had been looking for! Most impressive to me was how infrared science allows us to detect and catalog emotional traumas that reveal how we psychologically create our diseases and disharmony.

Infrared scanning makes quick, simple, advanced organ/gland energy observations that are decoded by our body's own 'organic language' to scientifically reveal an integrated, multi-dimensional view of our personal programming and functioning which is literally a scientific integration of our physical, emotional, mental and Spirit Life-force energy aspects.

Infrared scanning measures infrared heat from the body. The heat tells us where there is a density of electrons caused by resistance (drag) that causes heat and degeneration. This tells us where there is resistance in our electron energy flow patterns through specific electrical circuits that empower or disempower certain of our specific mental, emotional and physical functions.

Personal data from an infrared scan comes from all 253 organ/gland electrical circuits (connected energetically). The data reveals what, where and how organ/gland powers are being suppressed by trauma memory drag (which creates drag on expressing each specific circuit's power, function and purpose).

The validity of this organic system became instantly apparent to me when Joe did a quick one-minute scan on my girlfriend Arlene (before any significant dialogue between them had occurred) who happened to have spent that day scrubbing an unventilated bathroom with ammonia. After scanning her face and looking at the numbers from her scan (which appeared on a computer screen) and then flipping through a few pages in a book, Joe turned to Arlene and said, "How did you get toxic poisoning from ammonia?"

This experience changed my life, because I knew instantly that for him to be able to decode such specific detailed insight so accurately and quickly, there had to be a highly organized *natural organic system*. This would be the only way a scientific technique could tap into and decode these subtle levels of processing and communication (energy-motion) between our *body, mind and Spirit Life-force energy* – almost immediately!

While I was still in Florida, and with this exciting discovery as my impetus, I began studying this science that reveals an *organ/gland language from infrared measurements*. And at some point, I was asked to work with my very first client who turned out to be one of my lifelong friends, Louise L. Hay. And within a few months, Louise invited me to Santa Monica, CA. where she began to introduce me to her circle of friends. I eventually moved there and spent five more years working with individual clients and perfecting my knowledge of this science of organ/gland energy flow and drag between organs and glands. I became more and more experienced with how a one-minute infrared scan could decode a client's energy flow patterns into the unconscious decisions responsible for programming the problems in their life. After being used to taking so long to find the basic information I needed to make what I thought at the time were accurate psychological assessments, the thought of having this capability with each of my clients within minutes was hard for me to believe, *but extremely inspiring!*

With this tool, I could now actually measure the un-cleared trauma memory (unconscious decisions) in my client's twenty-three organ/gland circuits with utmost precision! I learned that our organ/gland energies are like recording devices or energy receptors. When the electrical drag from trauma memory creates resistance in our organ/gland circuits of power, the Life-force energy flow we receive from our Spirit *decreases* in these systems. When we are *conscious* enough in the moment to *override our drag* to make a different choice (inspired from our Spirit's Love and Light), then the Life-force energy flow from our Spirit is increased in those circuits between our twenty-three organ/gland energy systems.

I soon reached the point where I was getting more clinical information from a one-minute scan than I had ever gotten from clients using traditional, psychological methods, after months or even years! This science provided a much deeper, clearer and more accurate insight into the *mental and emotional causes of problems* in our body and in our life in general. I use this insight to raise a client's consciousness to identify and correct the unconscious decisions and actions responsible for their disease, disorder, dysfunction, and degeneration which has been created from the drag on their energy needed to regenerate their energy systems.

Now I finally had the tools for understanding the full spectrum of our being, and for obtaining a completely integrated, scientific and organic view of who we are and how we function on all levels. I also learned the importance of the answering these questions: *How do we function energetically? Who are we as Spirit? Where do we focus our energy? When do we make conscious and unconscious decisions? Why are we motivated to act as we do? And finally, what do we create as a result of our decisions and actions, and how do we learn to create our solutions?*

The answers to these questions provide the clarity needed to see and understand our problems and formulate conscious solutions that eliminate unconsciously programmed problems. Without this clarity and understanding, we are not sufficiently capable of doing what is needed to align with the energetic Laws of Spirit and nature. These organ/gland Laws of energy shine light on the pathway toward achieving *regenerative action* by being clear enough in the moment to see what is energetically and consciously *real* and to act spontaneously in alignment with it.

Since 1987 I have focused exclusively on this organ/gland language to enlighten clients about the energetic nature of who they are as humans, and then to track (using infrared) their un-cleared trauma memory programming of their electrical energy flow patterns that create sub-optimal functioning. This science provides me with an energetic mirror image (from client's organ/gland energy flow patterns) that provides integrated messages for aligning their physical, emotional, mental and Spirit Life-force energy functioning, for regeneration rather than degeneration.

When clear mental concepts of ourselves (for how we're designed to function) align with how we really function energetically, we are empowered by consciously connecting to *who we really are as Spirit Life-force energy*. Following the rules that define these Laws of energy empowers our concepts and the enacting of our plans. How we conceptualize ourselves and focus our attention is extremely important, because *attention* is our primary instrument of creation. *What we focus on is what we create!*

When we are conscious of how life works, life is largely a matter of proper timing (or being able to do the 'right thing at the right time') with clarity directing us 'in our moments of power.' Evolution is all about evolving from *fear*-oriented survival to *love*-oriented *fulfillment*. Knowing which of these motives are driving us allows us to make more conscious decisions *motivated by Love and Light* (which creates our solutions) instead of making decisions *motivated by fear* (which creates our problems).

This consciousness can be arrived at by observing Life-force electrical *energy flow patterns* with infrared scanning, and then decoding them with the body's own innate organic language (used by our cellular bio-computer) that reveals how our regenerative/degenerative pathways are directing all our functions.

As you will learn in this book, the body's electrical system consists of *253 two-way circuits* (the binomial pairs or permutations of twenty-three systems).

These 253 circuits connect each of our *twenty-three organ/gland energy systems* with every other organ/gland energy system. This electrical grid powers our *twenty-three physical, emotional, mental and Spirit Life-force energy functions* that direct our plans and functions in life.

These circuits can be *measured* with infrared scanning and be *numerically configured* around the *constant* order of organ/gland importance for survival. Then we can *decode* these measurements for each organ/gland blocked function, so they *reveal what we are doing* that is creating specific patterns of blocked electrical energy flow (these are called 'uplinks') that are associated with specific diseases, dysfunctions and disorders.

By monitoring the flow of Spirit Life-force energy through our 253 circuits, 'The BodyTalker' infrared scanner provides us with an exceptional level of clarity and insight (scientific validation) that shows how our physical, emotional and mental functions, by design, do integrate with each other. This science is therefore an invaluable tool for those seeking personal enlightenment to consciously empower them to clearly see the energetic pathways that must be followed to fulfill their Spirit's divine intent (their Spirit's life purpose).

Consciousness is about enlightening our confusions so we don't reactively make *unconscious fear-oriented decisions* but instead make *conscious Reality oriented decisions* that direct conscious actions. We can learn to discipline ourselves to make clear, conscious, love/light-oriented decisions that seek energetic truth with pleasure, which when consistently followed will create whatever our Spirit desires. At this point we come to consciously know that no other real solutions even exist.

For the past 2000 years, we have lived in the Age of Pisces, also called the "Age of Belief," during which we followed masters who 'knew' (meaning they knew about the science of energetic Reality). Starting in 2012, we entered the Age of Aquarius where enlightenment is the keynote for knowing/living truth within *ourselves* in accordance with the Laws of Spirit Life-force energy. Living this truth sets us free from the drag of 'missing the mark' energetically – which is what separates us from our Spirit. This separation, or going against Spirit's true nature of Love and Light, is the true definition of 'sin' (which is an old archery term that means "missing the mark" in the center).

This book is for those who are committed to becoming clear about their lives and learning to express their clarity and truth so they can manifest their divine intent. I tell my clients that this energetically aligned pathway is the *'only road out of town'* because instead of *unconsciously* sabotaging themselves, they can *consciously* make choices to create solutions that serve their Spirit to perform their divine intent for their own personal power and grace.

KNOW THYSELF

Summary

How Humans Are Designed to Function

Humans are designed to function so they can *naturally regenerate. This occurs* when their concepts of energetic Reality actually align with energetic Reality as it exists in life – so they may learn to follow this alignment. In other words, when their *'map' matches the 'territory'* they travel, they can then learn better how to master the territory needed in order to find the regenerative Way of life!

> *Doing things the Way they are not designed*
> *to work...means they cannot work!*

> *Doing things the Way they are designed to work...*
> *means they can, will, and do work!*

When we do things the way they don't work, our system gives us messages (we call them symptoms) that tell us *how* we are creating our problems if we can decode our *symptoms* into our *messages*. These decoded messages tell us *how to create our elegant solutions* that prevent and eliminate our problems. This book is about decoding those hidden energetic messages in precisely the way our bodies were designed to communicate with us through our organs and glands. This is what we refer to as the 'language of the body.'

Life is an energy game that we all must play every day in every way (and play or do it very well) to get sufficient *points* with few enough *penalties* that we can still fulfill our Spirit's life (without being consumed by our dragons ways). But, if we don't *know* the game of energy (we are forced to play) and we don't *see* how the game of life works (with the Rules and our Tools) we can't *play* it so it *works for us.*

Our human design is quite simple to understand. Once the design is seen clearly in its integrated energetic format, this point of view becomes self-evident and undeniable. Then, at that point, operating in alignment with who we already are energetically becomes simple to see but *not necessarily easy to do*, because of old familiar habits of unconscious (dragon) memory.

Once we can consciously align with our organ/gland Spirit Life-forces of who we already are, we can stay connected to our present in each moment where our power is! We cannot do this if we still have the unconscious drag of *reactive* fears from earlier trauma memory triggered by current feeling associations. These put us into *time-warps* of our past that we relive in our present, which consume our present time and energy.

This book shows how our personal life happens daily according to how well our integrated organ/gland energetic systems are able to consciously process and perform their regenerative functions and avoid their defensive unconscious degenerative programming that creates their dysfunctions.

Chapter 1

Clarifying the Solutions to Human Problems

Consciousness is Clarity in Action

The twenty-first century began with the Year of the Dragon (in the Chinese calendar), which symbolizes getting rid of everything that no longer serves us in our life. It began a time of massive change in our world, challenging us to live *consciously* and align with the Laws of energetic Reality and our Spirit's divine intent to be effective and ful-filled at being who we really are – Spirit Life-force in physical form.

There are many challenges and stresses in our lives which require making changes to adapt to an increasingly changing environment. These challenges necessitate a more refined *personal clarity* in order to function effectively in our *moments of power* (a moment of power is the 'crunch time' in any game – when we either make or lose the 'shot'). We are all required to play this energy game of life daily as long as we are alive, and (like all games) there are no points for defense!

This means we must play offensively and proactively to win 'points.' When we 'take our shots' by speaking our truth (clearly, quickly and appropriately) this scores points without 'fouling.' ('Foul-ing' is about using our Life-force just to survive dysfunction that con-scious behavior would have prevented.)

Life is like basketball or football, in that no matter how good we are at 'defense,' defense alone does not create points to win the game and create sustainable solutions to solving our problems. When we view our life as 'surviving the problem' (for instance, if we think: "The other team has the ball – and I can't do anything about it because that's just the way it is."), we enable/maintain our problems by *accepting them.*

But if we are conscious enough to *not accept those triggered defensive thoughts* (from past memories) and we are then able to *focus* our attention on *getting the ball* (knowing our truth), and then get into position to *shoot the ball* (express our truth effectively) we are getting there. But, then the real points come from when we can speak our truth with the right dose of the right energy expressed at the right time within the usual one-second openings – and do it *without fouling* – which is when we will consistently make our 'points!'

So, our ability to play our game of life (for more points and fewer penalties) depends on our offensive or pro-active ability to *know the Rules* and *'show up'* with our organ/gland energy Tools to perceive and express our truth in our life. This comes down to knowing and following the Laws of energy – so the force of those Laws is *with you* (rather than being *against you*).

Playing 'offense' allows for *real regenerative solutions* by focusing on what creates the solutions that solve our problems and eliminate what is causing them, thus *preventing them from ever being created!*

In other words, in order to win the game of life, we must make conscious decisions that direct conscious actions aligned with the Laws of energy, so we flow with the *force* of those Laws to regenerate ourselves. Otherwise, if we *misalign* with the Laws of energy the flow of energy is against us – which degenerates our organ energies.

This means we must make clear, conscious decisions (in the moment). These decisions must then align with energetic Reality (as it really exists) or – we have confusion! We must take actions that align with the descriptive Laws/Rules of energy that are the foundation of physics and metaphysics (subtle energy).

In the end, it comes down to being able to live, perceive and perform by decisions that are instinctively and spontaneously aligned with our Spirit and the natural Laws of energy. So our only challenge is to become more conscious of our Spirit's Ways of Love and Light and learn to better follow them, moment by moment. This is what higher consciousness is all about – consciousness in the moment for energetic Reality so we can make regenerative decisions rather than degenerative ones.

Living without refinement in how we think and act, compared to living in *refined alignment* with the Laws of energy – is best portrayed by the problem encountered by physicists when they learned they could not use classical Newtonian physics to fly to the moon. It can't be done,

34

because classical physics concepts are *insufficiently refined energetically* to be able to define the subtle energetic reality that exists in space between the earth and the moon.

It wasn't until these *subtle levels of energy could be measured and accurately calculated mathematically* that science was clear enough about energetic Reality to be able to account for and accurately predict the gravitational effects on a beam of light needed to *pinpoint the exact location* where the moon would be when they got there!

The difference between *classical* and *quantum* mathematics is in their *conceptual ability to define* the more refined and subtle aspects of energetic Reality. It's all about the finer and finer differentiations of *energy from 'black and white' to sixteen trillion colors* (which comes from more and more subtle discriminations of perceptual observations of energy). The understanding of these subtle variations and finer discriminations have made electronics possible (as well as making possible the many advanced inventions such as high-definition television and space travel)! These advances give us more of what works, and less of what doesn't work in the world of modern electronics.

High-definition television is made possible through the use of cables containing gold, which is a refined, super-conductor of precise subtle energy. Analogously, for humans to have 'high-definition consciousness,' we need refined, precise discernment and processing of subtle energies which show up as personal power – when our consciousness becomes our superconductor of subtle energy!

As we see how the Laws work either *for us or against* us in the short and long term, we see the bigger picture of the *energy game* of life that every person is forced to play every day. How we play this energy game determines the outcomes in our health, body, business and relationships and everything in our lives. When we can learn to fly on automatic pilot guided by the Light of clarity about energetic Reality in our own personal life expressions, it inspires (or 'in-Spirit's' us), which regenerates our health while also creating a more meaningful and fulfilling existence.

> *Higher consciousness is the equivalent of personal clarity, effectiveness, efficiency and productivity that aligns with the Light (Ways of our Spirit). This allows us to make clear decisions more quickly because we can see the outcome of our decisions before we make them. When clear conscious forethought directs our actions in the moment, we avoid the stress and heartache of dysfunctional decisions creating continuous chaos in our life*

Living consciously enables us to process our life experiences in alignment with the Laws of energy (Reality), so our decisions align with their power, to create *regeneration* in our lives.

If we are not making healthy *aligned decisions* that regenerate, then we are making *misaligned decisions* of drag (homeostasis by drag) that degenerate and cause us to *go backward in circles*. This defensive strategy eventually manifests as symptoms (with messages) of physical mass or emotional matters. They result from blocked/unsolved trauma memory programming that creates an 'energy motion' (e 'motion'al) issue of perception and/or expression.

Over time the drag of trauma memory creates *mass* from the same programming that creates *matters*. These emotional matters manifest as physical organ/gland dysfunctions, which cause our physical health problems and are associated with very specific emotional dysfunctions which were usually programmed by specific types of trauma memory.

It takes consciousness to be *true to our Spirit* so that we may manifest the gifts of our divine intent to make our unique contributions to the world. Who we are consciously determines our potential for evolving our life, because only consciousness gives us a clear choice to manifest our Spirit's desires.

Consciousness gives us our *personal power* by speeding up our *processing time* which is determined by our ability to (1) *first clearly perceive* what's causing our problem, and (2) then *processing our knowing* of the cause quickly into effective actions that **eliminate our problem!** This is what true prevention is all about and what is required to stay 'ahead of the curve' – where all winners play to win.

The Problems We Don't Create ... We Don't Have!

Our most *basic solution* to human problems is first clearly seeing and understanding who we are as Spirit Life-force energy. Then, we can more clearly perceive and express each organ/gland's Spirit Life-force energy so our physical functioning is always supported by healthy emotional processing and mental programming that effectively operates all of the important and essential aspects of our lives.

Once we are clear about the nature of energetic Reality and how the energy game of life actually works, obviously we can play it better. Such clarity allows us to better observe the real life issues facing us, versus the ones that are not so real. We also begin to see how our problems come from the *confusions* of not seeing energetic Reality clearly.

Confusion (when our *concepts* don't *fuse* with Reality) limits our ability to effectively discern and conceive energetic Reality spontaneously, due to our unconsciously triggered and projected past imprinted trauma memory from our emotional programming.

How clearly we operate in alignment with energetic Reality determines whether we create *degenerative problems or regenerative solutions.* This is why the elegant solutions to any problem must always begin first by clearly seeing and understanding the problem at its *most causal levels of subtle energy* (memory) programming of our unconscious decisions.

Once we're aware of our subtle, unconscious, causal decisions, we can then see how our survival programming is creating a *drag on our Spirit Life-force perceptions and expressions* of our personal reality! In order to override this powerful unconscious programming, we must be conscious enough in the *moment of our decision* to make a Spirit choice. Understanding our body's language clarifies our choices so we can be extremely clear about what we need to do and not do to regenerate our Life-force.

Only when we become conscious of our unconscious decisions can we gain control over our old programmed decision patterns. Our ability to *consciously* get ahead of our old familiar *unconscious* decisions *in the moment* enables us to direct our actions *in the present* from the present – rather than from our past. If our past association triggers from reactive trauma memory *remain in unconscious control*, they will continue to make decisions that direct our life *for us.*

37

Once we realize where, when and how we are expressing the drag on our Life-force energy flow, we can catch ourselves *consciously before* our triggered unconscious memory reactivates our dragon's decisions for us. We can then consciously *imprint new decision-making patterns* and habits (actual physical, synaptic changes from learning) for new decisions and actions that *update our memory banks* with conscious, regenerative expressions that direct our life and future.

As we begin to see ourselves from this subtle energy point of view, our personal insights and consciousness become greatly refined, expanded and clarified beyond the visible rainbow of our third-dimensional perspectives (basis of most traditional health practices). With higher consciousness we gain a much more *complete and integrated view* of the Reality of 'Who we are and how we function, energetically.'

What is the 'Drag' on Our Spirit's Life-force Energy Flow?

When our Spirit Life-force energy flow is blocked by trauma memory programming, health problems result. This is because the energy flow to and from our organs and glands is short-circuited when our decisions are being made by triggered unconscious trauma memory. This process is clearly revealed through infrared scanning of our natural circuits of electrical (electrons) energy flow patterns. When we can see our programmed blocks which act as a 'drag' on our Spirit Life-force energy flow, we can *then* choose to perform more functional actions for better outcomes by making *clearer decisions quicker.*

Like the mythical dragons that stand as fierce guardians at the entrance to important buildings, the 'drag' on Spirit Life-force energy from trauma memory acts as a guardian or survival mechanism that attempts to protect us from whatever triggers our *trauma memory.* These electrical 'drags' on our Spirit Life-force energy reactively project our past decisions (our trauma memory) onto our present. This causes us to unconsciously perceive and act (in our present) as though our present was the *same as our past* (which is almost never true)!

Although such perceptions may not be real, our projected dragon memory makes unconscious decisions spontaneously *as if* they were real in the present (the same as our past trauma or triggered memory) *unless* we consciously override our reactive decisions in our moments of power.

Big 'R' *Reality* as it exists in the *present* and *future* does not relate to the *dragon's reality,* because the dragon's reality is a triggered past memory of trauma. This is why it often distorts everything sometimes because its orientation comes from a past *there and then* perspective about what is actually present *here and now.*

The dragon makes up its own defensive rules that are based on knowing how to use **confusion** and **deception** to **manipulate** others with *fear* and *force* (which defines the negative rules – or the ways of the dragon). And so, the dragon puts a lot of focus into learning to *act real* without really *being real,* because that's how deception gives the dragon its power. It doesn't want to be real. It wants to sell others on its acting out a part to *appear real* in order to get you to ***buy whatever it is selling!***

If we buy what the dragon is selling, we then *own* the drag! Then if we *own* the drag, we've got to *store* the drag, and pay the *cost of the storage* on the drag, while also having to *deal with the effects* of the drag on our life and body … ***every day of our life!***

Our dragons are designed for *short-term solutions,* but over time they create *long-term problems.* When defensive dragon fears control our behavior, our blocked organ/gland energy creates *disease, disorder, dysfunction* and *degeneration.* Inappropriate fears limit our ability to clearly discern our *perceptions* and effectively *express* our truth with power.

Consciousness is about whether or not we can get ahead of our triggered unconscious programs. That decision is probably made *within a thousandth of a second from the stimulus.* This is the *precise moment* when you decide *to be* (which is to use our organ/gland energy function to perceive and express its particular energy), or *not to be* (which is to use the ways of 'drag' to endure and survive by *not* using our true organ/gland perceptions and expressions, *as if* we had no choice or power to change or escape our situation). These kinds of decisions over time ultimately lead to our dysfunction and degeneration.

On the other hand, our Spirit's strategy is to align what we *see* and *feel* with what we *say* and *do,* and notice who makes us feel safe and worthy of love. We will pay special attention to those who continuously treat us with respectful actions that are always clear, quick and appropriate with honor for Love and Light.

Our emotional powers and abilities come directly from our ability to consciously perceive, connect with, and effectively express our true feelings. This provides for clear perceptual inputs and expressive outputs. This is what true transparency is all about!

This frees our energy circuits to flow without blocks (that restrict or drag) on our refined perceptions and effective creative expressions. Consciousness clearings (or *ah ha's*) in our circuits often cause the body to experience a spontaneous jerking motor response. This is called an ideo-motor response or *idea*-motor response at the very moment of insight. This is something we have all likely experienced at some point – and even exclaimed: *"Ah ha!"* This connection between our *conscious mind* and our *unconscious knowing* is part of our actual enlightening experience of *becoming more fully conscious.*

Our organ/gland energy flow is *blocked* when present circumstances *trigger* past associated memories of not feeling safe or able to perceive and express our truth. *Not feeling safe* blocks the flow of Life-force energy that connects our circuits to give us personal power. These unconscious triggered reactions disconnect us from our Spirit's Life-force energy in order to *counterbalance* not feeling safe or being able to perceive or express our Spirit's truth. (This happens when we have been traumatized and disconnected in order to suppress the expression of how we really feel emotionally.)

We free our Self of these electrical 'drags' or energy blocks, by being *conscious enough in the moment* of our triggered r*eactive programming* to *take a deep breath* (instead of reacting), and allow other people's Spirits to feel safe (from our reacting) and free to express their truth. Only this allows for *productive conversing* of different views that allows Spirits to get smarter by revealing what does not align with energetic Reality. By doing this consistently we become more able to see and process our own blocked expressions of 'drag' on our Spirit Life-force energy flow much more effectively and productively.

To summarize, the *only elegant solution to human problems* is being conscious enough to have the ability to easily, naturally and instinctively respond to life with *conscious decisions* based on clear, spontaneous perceptions of Reality that direct our actions to harmoniously align with the Laws of Spirit and nature.

Clarity in our view of these natural Laws when integrated into our conscious decisions – directs our actions and enables us to *foresee the consequences of our choices before they happen,* and thus allows us to make *wiser decisions quicker.* This naturally gives us more conscious control over what we create in our life and our body, as well as in our relationships and business.

Otherwise, whatever *interferes* with our ability to make clear, quick and appropriate decisions, choices and actions *diminishes* our functioning ability and *increases* the creation of havoc in our lives and bodies!

When we can *sustain clear conscious perceptions, decisions and actions consistently* enough, we create real, long-term solutions to our problems because our actions align with the Laws of our Spirit and nature.

This results in our being healthier as well as more efficient, effective and productive as human beings. In the long term, this is *our pathway to global human solutions* because our clarity for our personal subtle energetic Reality allows us to solve our human problems!

When we make clearer, more effective decisions quicker and can perform our truth clearly, quickly and appropriately, we can then create the fulfillment of our solutions – which further enlivens and regenerates our cells, bodies and lives to become more of Who we really are as Spirit.

The 'Living in a Bubble' Exception

As we can imagine, being clear, quick and appropriate in our actions creates more balanced, centered feelings within our being. This allows us to extend our Spirit's feelings of Love and peace with its Light of truth for the Laws to all Spirits around us which makes everyone feel more fulfilled and connected.

When we act more in alignment and harmony with the Laws of energy and the Ways of Spirit that define how the energies of our bodies and lives really work, there is *less resistance* to the natural energetic flow of life than when we act *against* the force of these natural Laws and Ways of energy flowing.

However, there is one exception to this rule. When a group of people *act together out of alignment* with certain Laws of Spirit and nature (by agreeing on certain *distortions of truth about Reality*) this creates *mutual agreement for distortion.* It creates a *distorted consensus* to make a thing *look real that is not real.*

A case in point is when people thought the earth was flat, because they had a *distorted consensus of agreement* with a flat world 'bubble' view; and the 'round world Truth' was dangerous even to think, discuss or express (even though that view accurately aligned with energetic Reality).

This is an *illusion* created from a *delusion* about what is real. *It turns 'Real' into what is 'not real'* and what is 'not real' into what is 'real' (for those in the bubble – 'not real' is defined as a bubble perception which is true only in the bubble world). If this is the case, what is really Real (in terms of energetic Reality) will be ridiculed and seem completely out of line to the bubble reality consciousness.

Another prime example in the health field is where the general public is often led to believe in something that later turns out to be untrue. Eating eggs was initially considered to be *very good.* Then it was considered *very unhealthy* – and now it is considered *healthy again.*

Vitamin E, once considered to be *useless,* now is considered *essential. Nothing actually changed in energetic Reality* except our own *perception* of what is Real.

Consequently, we live in a very confused world, with collective distortions compounded with individual distortions, amidst tremendous accelerating changes in knowledge, insight, information and technology. Now we are forced to adapt and accommodate very quickly just to keep up. To do this in a healthy, balanced way, we must consistently make clear, quick, effective decisions based on clear conceptual observations and understandings of energetic Reality.

However, *first* we must be as clear and conscious as possible about how the mysterious human organ/gland computer really works. Otherwise our organ/gland systems can be unconsciously programmed by our old past trauma memory software, so that we reactively run our entire life and body from our projected unconscious decisions of past trauma memory programming.

The organ/gland concept gives us our natural structure and framework for consciousness about who we are and how we function as *energy systems* designed to help us clarify our problems so we may create more elegant solutions that inspire and fulfill us.

Socrates said, "Know thyself," because nothing is more important for us to know than our *Whole, Spirit 'Self'!* Knowing our true Self in terms of how we are designed to function is extremely important in order for us to function consciously in how we use our own personal hardware and software energetically. Getting to really know our human computer is not easy (or even possible) when one has only a physical view (which is only 1/88th of our energetic Reality) and rudimentary understanding of the much bigger subtle energy picture of Reality!

The confusion that results from being limited to mere physical understanding may be our greatest human confusion problem at this time. This creates confusion, because our physiological view of who we are is much too limited to ever be able to see and know our whole, integrated, energetic Self we are.

The solutions to our problems can never be any better than the clarity of our concepts for understanding what is creating our problems. If we cannot see clearly who we are and how we function, we can never be sufficiently clear to make the decisions and take the actions needed to create our real solutions. Thus, our clarity for the structure and function of our personal mind/brain/body computer is extremely important!

Also, our conscious *conceptual* model of who we are and how we function must align with energetic Reality in order to integrate with our basic energetic design that was set at conception (when our twenty-three chromosomal light-body male energies from our father came together with the twenty-three chromosomal light-body female energies from our mother).

These twenty-three double helix pairs of chromosomes are the memory banks at the nucleus of our original cell of conception that give us the structure that directs all our functions. This original cell provides our holographically programmed memory (genetic planning mechanism) that directs our Life-force energy flow to create twenty-three organ/gland energy/body systems that predispose us to unconsciously function in the same format as our original chromosomal (light-body) programming.

Our Chromosomal Model for Personal Reality

Our chromosomal light-body computer programs our dense-body energy to follow our original design. That design is a twenty-three base system format of twenty-three physical organs and glands with twenty-three emotional functions and twenty-three mental plans that program our twenty-three Spirit Life-force organ/gland energy systems (100% of *who we are physically, emotionally and mentally*).

Our original cell of conception duplicates and divides itself over 280 days of gestation to create our twenty-three organ/gland energy systems directed by a light-body hologram of organ structures and functions in the nucleus of our original cell within the twenty-three pairs of our chromosomal memory.

Our powers and problems are determined by whether our energy *drags or flows* through our *253* organ/gland energy circuits that connect our twenty-three Spirit Life-force physical, emotional and mental energy functions.

Just as in the game of basketball, *defense is where you make no points* and *offense is where you make points.* Our Life-force energy can either be programmed by *clear conscious mental concepts or by confused unconscious trauma memory* that can be reactively triggered to direct our performance *defensively* from past memory. Having clear concepts aligned with Reality, means we can direct our Life-force energy *offensively* (pro-actively for energetic points) by using our personal power to create our elegant solutions.

Our *issues* end up in our *tissues* if they are not energetically cleared. By scientifically tracking our energy flow patterns and decoding them with our natural organ/gland energetic language, we can clearly see the 'drag' on each of our blocked 253 circuits that connect our twenty-three organs and glands. This observation reveals our developing *tissues* that are subject to health problems and their corresponding emotional *issues* that are blocking our subtle energy flow and stealing our personal power.

These problems exist first at the Spirit Life-force energy level when we are directed by decisions and actions primarily motivated by *fear*. After awhile these defensive dragon patterns manifest into denser and denser energy (because that's what drag is designed to do over time). This process is what we call *aging*. But the real issue causing this confused direction of energy is our triggered, unconscious decisions that are projected into our moments of power. This is what contributes to the blocked or semi-blocked expression of each organ and gland circuit.

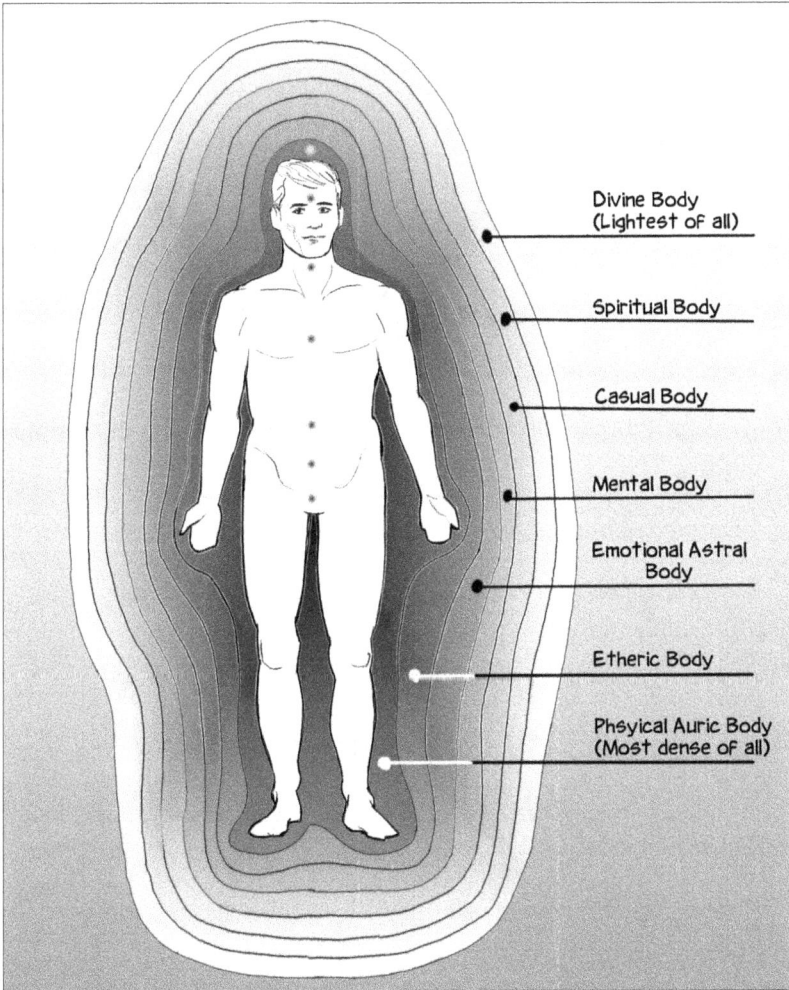

Auric levels

Organ/Gland; Physical Action, Emotional Function, Mental Plan, and Spirit Purpose

Each of our organ/gland energies has physical *actions* driven by emotional feeling *functions* following a conscious or unconscious mental *plan* to ideally fulfill its Spirit Life-Force energy *purpose*. The following one liner 'organ/gland energy descriptors' introduce you to the primal essence of each of your Spirit Life-force organ/gland energies that constitute your entire 'organ/gland language':

1. Thymus: ***protecting*** by appropriate aggression for safety, trust and independence

2. Heart: ***synchronizing*** with harmony to feel worthy of love

3. Colon: ***detoxifying*** by eliminating what we hate to avoid toxicity

4. Stomach: ***digesting*** what is nurturing to sustain happiness

5. Anterior Pituitary: ***directing*** from clear observation to master our Life-force

6. Liver: ***transmuting*** by focused expectation to create rejuvenation

7. Lungs: ***exchanging*** prana/oxygen to refresh Life-force by breathing into challenges

8. Sex Organs: ***connecting*** through attraction to create and reproduce

9. Bones and Muscles: ***moving*** to approach pleasure and avoid pain

10. Thyroid: ***metabolizing*** anxiety into action to correct personal injustice

11. Veins/Arteries: ***circulating*** against restrictions to participate in the games of life

12. Brain/Nervous System: ***electrifying*** circuits to simplify confused complications

13. Adrenals: ***equalizing*** by equal and opposite pressure with courage, capability and pride

14. Mind: ***analyzing*** unknowns by wondering how they reveal order to provide serenity

15. Hypothalamus: *evaluating* by sensory input to create results by clear communication

16. Kidneys: *filtering* by feeling toxic emotional situations and screening them out of life

17/18. Endocrine System: *balancing* for homeostasis in trauma by conserving Life-force energy

19. Skin: *demarcating* identity by defining, defending and expressing our true Self

20. Pancreas: *locating* our divine intent by expressing and following our truth

21. Posterior-Pituitary: *hydrolyzing* to cleanse our losses and free us from being stuck in grief

22. Parathyroid: *experiencing* decisiveness for what we really do and don't want

23. Spleen: *rejecting* antagonism in order to avoid regret from feeling disrespected

24. Lymph: *clarifying* what is acceptable by knowing and understanding energetic Reality

Blockages from trauma memories are the cause of our problems. It is how our issues show up in our tissues. With this organ/gland language and infrared scanning, we can actually see where and how our Life-force energy *issues* exist at the subtle emotional-causal levels of energy flow. By making conscious decisions we can prevent problems years before they manifest physically in our *tissues*.

Fear-motivated decisions create emotional dysfunctions in our *life* that manifest as physical dysfunctions in our *body*. Our body is the final resting place for the physical manifestations of these dysfunctions we call 'symptoms,' which all have 'solution messages' coded within them. Consistent blockage of particular circuits over a sustained period of time creates disorders, dysfunction, disease and degeneration in the energies of our life, body, business and relationships.

Each organ and gland has its own *unique vibratory energy* designed to perform specific physical, emotional, mental and Spirit Life-force energy *functions* (outlined in the chapters ahead). When we are able to see how we operate energetically, we can then learn to practice functioning much more effectively, efficiently and productively in our life by knowing and following the Rules of Reality around who we are energetically and how we are designed to function in order to regenerate and sustain our Life-force energy.

We can then more easily see and understand how to be more conscious of what input creates what outcome depending on what decisions we make in the moment. As we become more conscious of the Law and ways of energy we reach the point where we can see the outcome *before* we make our decisions so we can *choose from a sense of consciousness* for the Laws of energy that define how things work.

When we live in harmony with the Laws of energy, our body is energized with health! We also feel safe and worthy of love, and able to perceive and express our true emotional feelings with a loving intent that connects with our truth and regenerates feelings of happiness and fulfillment.

Unclear decisions (resulting from inadequate foresight) create confusion in our lives that causes us to feel fear. This results in a cycle of reactive decisions, chaos, trauma and further confusion in our lives. Repeating these familiar self-destructive decisions increases the 'drag' on our system and perpetuates dysfunctional patterns of behavior that accelerates fatigue (which ages and diminishes our quality of life).

One of the greatest challenges facing human beings is being able to consciously realize that only through actions of Love directed by the Light of truth (alignment with the Spiritual and natural Laws of energy) can we find real solutions to human problems. This is how consciousness becomes the only elegant solution to human problems, because only consciousness gives us a *conscious choice* to solve our own problems by functioning further 'ahead of the curve.' Clearer and quicker decision-making is consciousness in action!

[This basic message (operating clearer and quicker ahead of the curve) will be repeated often in this book, because it pertains to almost everything in terms of being able to claim our power and perform it quicker to create points!]

The reason this kind of positive energetic performance gets points is because when you do it energetically right you will have what, in the movies, is called 'believability' (which is the only thing that gives anyone any power in *life* or on the *screen*). That's because *if nobody believes you, you don't have any power!* Therefore, consciousness is naturally the first priority for all human Spirits who truly seek to live in the Ways that work to enhance our *regeneration* and diminish our *degeneration* by simply learning to effectively and productively perform our innate powers so they can solve most of our human problems.

KNOW THYSELF

Chapter 2

Enlightening Your Pathway to Conscious Power

What's the Matter?

We humans are designed to *evolve* from a *fear-based consciousness of survival* (directed by past trauma memory) – to a *Love/Light Reality-based consciousness* for the fulfillment of our divine intent as our gift to the world. We are designed to do this by using clear conscious concepts to direct our actions to create and perform our solutions that prevent and eliminate our problems.

'Drag' (from trauma/fear memory) on this process of functional evolvement creates all our matters!

To evolve, we must become clear, quickly enough to be sufficiently conscious in our moments of power to override triggered, unconsciously projected past memory of dysfunctional decisions, and be able to function ahead of the curve so we are always moving forward and seldom moving backward in our life. When we can do this consciously and keep ahead of our old patterns with new decisions, we then imprint new memory of new behaviors that we add to our performance of our new functional decision-making patterns that then override old dysfunctional habits.

Dysfunctional decisions are reactively triggered when we consciously or unconsciously associate an earlier experience in our past with a similar feeling in our present. Consciously recognizing our Spirit's truth (what is naturally revealed to us in every one of circuits when they are not blocked) in the moment allows us to consciously choose what aligns, harmonizes and regenerates our organ/gland Spirit Life-force energy. This is what consciousness, regeneration and fulfillment are about.

The only real solution to human problems is having sufficient consciousness, soon enough, to align our decisions and actions with the regenerative Laws of energy, so the force of those Laws gives us our personal power to create our elegant solutions that come from following our Spirit's Ways.

These Laws of energy scientifically amount to measurements and observations that show how *three simple elements* of Reality connect and operate together at *different levels of density,* which can be conceived of as *mass, energy* and *concept.* This conception of energetic Reality is the basis of Einstein's formula ($E=MC^2$) that shows mathematically how energy is transferred into mass or how our unconscious memory (imprinted energy) is transferred into our symptoms and problems. This *clarity* solves many so-called *mysteries* about where many health issues and life problems come from, by suddenly making their origins self-evident and undeniable.

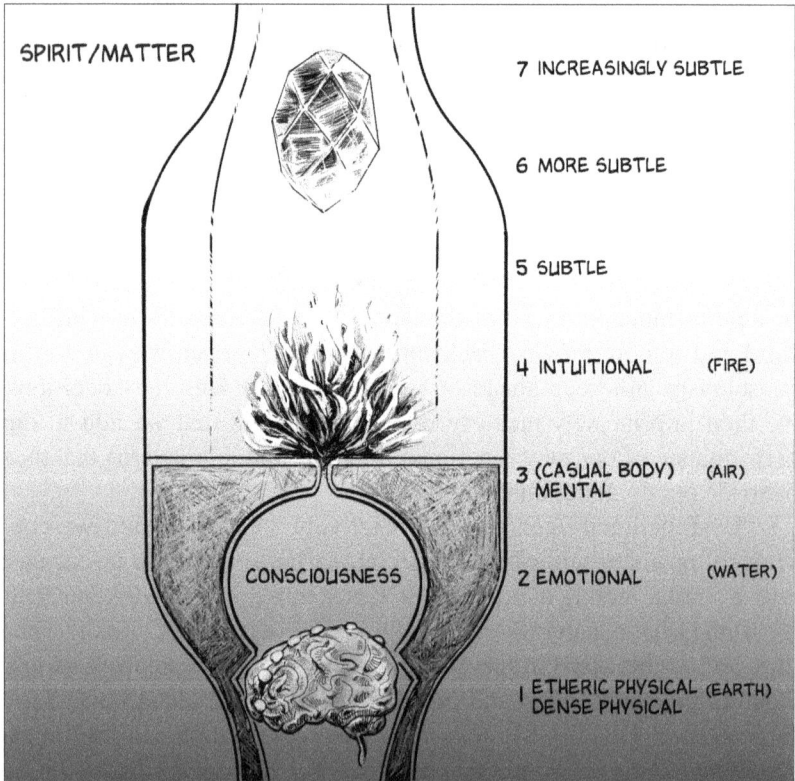

The illustration above shows the range of human energy at different levels of density and consciousness. Human energy connects through our chakras to our physical, emotional, mental and Spirit Life-force energy body. In the language of astrology, these different levels are called Fire, Air, Water and Earth. *(Special thanks to my friend Diane Magel, the airbrush artist who painted this for me when I taught my first consciousness class at Boise State University in 1978. This image was redrawn, for black and white print, by Bora Orcal.)*

A critical factor is in knowing when our Life-force energy is flowing *'North'* (being directed by our Spirit's Life-force in a productive and regenerative Way) versus when our Life-force energy is flowing 'South' (being directed by fear and the defensive ways of drag that degenerate us).

In the energetic game of life there are *no points for defense!* Defense is degenerative in nature because it achieves homeostasis by drag counterbalancing drag. This drag (over time) is our *problem* that we use to endure and survive what is not acceptable to our Spirit (because it does not harmonize with our Spirit's Ways/Laws that create solutions).

This degenerates as well as ages our organs and glands over the long term. The only way to achieve regenerative homeostasis is to create solutions that allow us to *not have to focus our energy on surviving our problems*. We do this by living in alignment with the regenerative Ways of our Spirit's Life-force that define the natural Laws of organ/gland energy that create our Spirit's elegant solutions.

Clarity of consciousness directed by *concepts* that align with Reality as it exists energetically determines our ability to direct our Spirit Life-force *energy* so we can create regenerative health and avoid degenerative problems. Physical symptoms are the effects of *mass* from 'drag' on Spirit Life-force energy flow manifesting as disease, disorder and dysfunction (like sand flowing around an obstacle in a stream). Over time, this defensive practice of living in drag eventually manifests as *masses* from unexpressed emotional *matters*. (This is where the age old question, "What's the matter?" stems from.)

Dr. Elmer Green (a professional associate of mine) was one of the earliest pioneers to work with humans at their subtle energy levels, and he was soon faced with the need to properly describe our Spirit energy conceptually. So he explained that 'Spirit' energy could be thought of as being part of a spectrum of energy. He said, "Spirit is the finest form of mass and mass is the densest form of Spirit."

Both of these concepts are true – because ***everything is energy*** – which means that energetic Reality is a continuum of different levels of energy density. Spirit Life-force is our most subtle energy and can be programmed by our past unconscious trauma memory or our present consciousness of energetic Reality.

In his famous formula, Einstein explains how we create our problems. ($E=MC^2$) shows how *Energy = Mass* times the *Constant* speed of light squared. In humans this formula translates into how trauma memory *(energy)* transfers into symptoms *(mass)* as the differential between energetic Reality *(as a constant)* – and how that *'squares'* with *our conscious view of energetic Reality.*

So, it follows that the clarity or confusion of our mental concepts (C) programs our Life-force energy (E) into our mass (M). This applies to our body, as well as the matters (problems) of our lives. In energetic Reality this creation happens exactly the way Einstein explains this process.

This *discrepancy* between *energetic Reality* and our *perceptual view of energetic Reality* spins energy backward and manifests as *symptoms with messages* that reveal our elegant solutions. Decoding these unique personal messages from the psycho-biophysics of this process explains how we transfer our *energy* (memory) into *mass* (symptoms/ problems) or in other words how our *trauma memory* becomes our third-dimensional, *visible symptoms and problems.*

Since all our memories are **only** a recording of Reality as we perceived it to be at the time of our memory, our memories by their very nature are usually distorted perceptions of energetic Reality. In other words, what happens is that when our dragon takes over we often unconsciously perceive reality **now** as being **the same** as our projected reality was perceived to be **then**.

Life being a continuum of different levels of human energy, Einstein's formula clearly explains how our triggered *unconscious* (E) energy (past trauma memory) associates with present time experiences. This explains why we reactively project our associations into *subconscious* perceptions of confused distortions of present Reality. 'Consciousness squared' (C^2) – the difference between our past and our present or what is real and what is unreal – manifests our symptoms as the distortions between 'big "R" Reality' and 'little "r" reality.' This distorted perception influences our decisions and directs our actions to create our *unconscious* emotional and physical effects that manifest as our personal problems and dysfunctions (M).

Electrical 'drag' (on Spirit Life-force energy flow) from 'trauma memory' is programmed to trigger and *project past associated memory into our present*, because these are the protective ways of the dragon doing its job. And since the dragon's primary job is protection motivated by fear, then living in fear about survival makes the dragon (trauma memory) feel useful and happy because it is doing what it is designed to do: *trigger, project and re-live old fear/trauma memory.*

However, remember our memories are *only* recorded perceptions of our past. Therefore, it is essential to have conscious awareness of how we are programmed to project re-lives of our past into our present and future, in order to be able to avoid repeating our past traumas. Lack of awareness for certain of our projected distortions causes our present experiences to get unconsciously morphed into time-warped perceptions from our past traumas that we unconsciously live out as our present dramas!

Only clear, conscious processing in the present moment can get us out of being in a degenerative cycle where we are unconsciously controlled and directed by past defensive, degenerative survival memory, which prevents us from being free to be Who we are as our Spirit's Life force.

Mass represents the symptomatic effect end of the energy spectrum, which is where effects manifest in our body physically, in our business monetarily, and in our relationships emotionally. All these effects come from either our conscious or our unconscious decisions that are directing our life and actions. In other words, dysfunctional physical symptoms are manifestations of confused emotional processing and mental/conceptual thinking or memory that programs our Life-force organ/gland energies to do (or not do) what creates our problems and our solutions.

Our Spirit's Life-force energy is our energetic Source of life! Therefore, consciously getting how specific past dysfunctional trauma programming is unconsciously making decisions for us in the present is how we evolve. We can do this by seeing what, when and how we can make new choices that shift our focus from creating our problems to spontaneously focusing on and performing what creates our solutions.

Winning the Energy Game (LIFE) We All Must Play Every Day

The creation of anything comes from maintaining a sufficient focus of attention on what it takes to manifest that creation over an adequate period of time to bring our creation to fruition. When we realize that our focused conscious attention is actually what creates whatever negative or positive thing we focus on, then we can learn to consciously focus our attention on aligning our decisions and/or actions with the natural Laws and our Spirit's Ways. Only then can we create solutions that eliminate our problems.

In other words, if we can't focus on something long enough and clearly enough, we cannot create it. When we do focus our attention on something long enough, we will create it (negative or positive).

A laser beam provides the perfect analogy for how this dynamic principle works. A laser beam is created by using a ruby to focus coherent light and when this light is intensified with power and directed toward opposing mirrors, the laser beam at a certain point of intensity breaks through one of the opposing mirrors. [See "Ideology" Dichotomy – The Secret of SAF: Scogna: 1986.]

When this focused coherent light finally breaks through the opposition, it can pierce steel and travels for light years. Analogously, when we focus coherent attention on anything long enough, we will ultimately create coherent refinements of clarity that allow us to walk the narrow straight path of alignment to deliver the right dose of the right energy to the right place at the right time. This is how we align with the Ways/Laws of subtle energy where all creation begins in that invisible subtle energy field beyond the visible 'rainbow.'

We are all 'starring' in our own personal movie called 'Our Life' that is always being filmed in our memory! Performing our role so it scores points is determined by how we deliver/perform our lines. Points in movies are about believability, which is determined by our ability to perform our scenes with a connected presence with what we really think and feel. This connection with our truth is best delivered with a 'Mona Lisa smile,' a loving intent and a quest for the truth in a conversational tone of voice.

When this *delivery* is timed and synchronized into consistent alignment with our body language – we show up as being spontaneous, clear quick and appropriate – which makes us *believable*. This defines personal power! When we do this consistently, this is what brings home the *points* for our performances in our life's movie. It's all about our ability to give our best performance of our truth... or *not!*

Life is like the movie business – *only two things matter – great scenes* and *bad scenes*. To make a movie work, we need *more* great scenes and *no* bad scenes (or at least fewer bad scenes)!

A bad scene is when we *inappropriately* time-warp from our *here/ now* to our *there/then* being projected from triggered associations with past memory which scripts and directs our present scenes from misaligned associations with our past. When we unconsciously do this, we empower our dragons to disconnect us even more from our Spirit's twenty-three personal powers. When effectively used, these are the same powers that provide us with all our real solutions.

Dragon solutions are never about providing us with long-term solutions – so they provide short-term solutions that *perpetuate* our problems and eliminate the possibility of ever being able to create our *long-term elegant solutions!*

Only when we start performing more believable and effective scenes in our life's movie, through our own consistent, conscious performances, do we learn to turn the *bad scenes* in our life into *great scenes* that effectively and *believably express our Spirit's truth in our moments of power.*

However, just learning our lines is not enough (nobody ever got an academy award just for knowing their lines). Personal power is all about how well we **perform** our lines in our moments of truth. This power is what really makes the **big difference**. In fact, how clearly and quickly we perceive a clear connection with our organ/gland feelings and express them, determines the believability of our deliveries and our personal power for everything we do in life!

Sustaining our personal power is about maintaining an offensive (pro-active) regenerative homeostatic balance by first being able to process input clearly at the same rate it is being received (i.e., at the speed of light – or instantly and spontaneously). If we can't do this, we have unprocessed input that may critically relate to some aspect of Reality we are trying to clearly figure out in order to get what we want.

If we receive input at the speed of light, we must ideally be able to process our true response clearly, consciously and **spontaneously** to be truly enlightened in that moment. On the street this is called *being real* or showing up. It is also very believable and therefore it sells movie tickets – especially interest in our own life's movie – which then inspires us even more to show up more in and for our own life.

So, 'being real' means clearly processing and delivering accurate reflections of energetic Reality spontaneously and consciously in the moment received from our subtle organ/gland feeling messages. To do this *clear, quick processing consistently,* we must operate from clear concepts in our mind that align perfectly with Reality as it exists energetically – *to predict and play the energy game of life so it works!*

Once we've mastered the ability to consciously focus our attention on the Ways of energetic Reality (that define our Spirit's Ways) we begin to experience feelings of personal power from being more aligned with our true Self, so *the forces of the Laws of energy are with us.* This makes us more able to consciously process (perceive and express) our life's issues more clearly, quickly and appropriately.

Doing this greatly reduces our confusions caused by using concepts that do not *fuse* with energetic Reality or the Laws/Ways of energy – to try to create harmony and regeneration. We cannot regenerate if we cannot *'get it together.'* This was a term popularized by the 'hippies.' (It's what I call their 'second commandment' that is necessary for creating real harmony and regeneration, *after* following their 'first commandment' for fulfilling our divine intent, which is to *'get real.'*)

'Get real' was the hippies' first commandment, because without *getting real* we can't *get it together,* because we'll always be consumed by the experience of confusion from being unreal. Our con-fusions are always created by the Reality gap between our perceptions, and how Reality actually exists energetically.

Personal power is about *eliminating the differential* between what we *think* is real and what we *know* is Real (Laws/Ways of energy), so our *thinking* is based on what we *know* – not what we *think*. We do this by learning to think in concepts that fuse and align with how energy actually works by the Laws of physics and meta-physics. Those who *know* don't have to *think* (except about what they *know*).

Hypothetical constructs are an essential backbone of the scientific research process. *They are made up constructs* (hypothetical – which are best guesses) that are mostly incomplete. This is because they are 'maps that don't necessarily fit the territory' – and that is why they are called 'hypothetical.' Science uses them (for lack of anything better) as a starting point to try to decipher and attain more refined clarity about the energetic Reality being researched.

The scientific method leaves us with no other choice, so using hypo-thetical constructs is not the problem. The problem is confusing a hy-pothetical for Reality by those who read the information later as if it was based entirely on *fact rather than a hypothetical construct.*

Many examples of this exist in our present day health system where things were thought to be one way and later proven to be another way (e.g., eggs are bad ... no, now they're good). Personal examples are when things happen in life where we think they are one way, when in reality they turn out to be a completely different way when clarified by more refining and defining concepts that clarify the subtle aspects of energetic Reality.

Energetic Reality is everything and it includes all the connections within us as well as connections with others. Some famous research in physics has shown conclusively that the experiment cannot be sepa-rated from the *experimenter*. Theoretical physicist, Werner Heisenberg, formulated the original argument and published it in 1927. The for-mulation became known as the "Heisenberg Uncertainty Principle." What this means is that whatever is happening is always an interac-tion between ourselves and others – because we are all energetically connected.

The real question is, do we consciously perceive and conceptual-ize the bigger unconscious subtle energy picture of energetic Reality? Is our mind conceptually clear enough to see ahead of our unconscious curves in our moments of power where our decisions are made? If not, we will continue to act in *default* by re-enacting memories of our past dysfunctions as our default decisions in our present life!

Of course the dragon would love us to believe that memory from our past can effectively serve us in our present – because dragons are memory that can only operate defensively by projecting, in order to protect, survive and endure what we can't change or escape. This unconscious reactive projecting (what we call 'time-warping') of our past memory that becomes triggered into our present experiences 'as if' they were real and true, is what dragons do continuously, every chance they get, when we are not conscious of what they are doing and don't get ahead of them!

Dragons will sell you anything you'll buy. And if you buy it, they will use that to justify how 'real' it is because you bought it! But what else is a dragon to do? Since defensive energy can only be and think defensively (backward thinking). So, the dragon's bottom line game is all about enduring and surviving without 'being Real.'

In other words, dragons are defensive by nature and only capable of dragon trust. (Dragon trust is defined as: "You can't trust anybody, anytime, about anything, ever!") This is why dragons only feel safe by looking out at the world defensively (to avoid recurrences of past traumas). Dragons do not trust the thought of ever feeling 'safe and worthy of love.' And yet this is required in real love or we can't feel and be safe enough to open the passage within to our Spirit world of loving acceptance for the Light of Truth.

A major misconception about the Laws of Reality is the idea that *there is no Reality,* but rather: *"We all just have our own unique views of reality* and *that's all there is!"* Even though it is true that we all have our individual *'little r'* realities, it does not mean there is no *'Big R' Reality'!* If there was no 'Big R' energetic Reality, there would be no order. The Universe would be in chaos and disorder (and there is less and less evidence for that being true).

This is because the larger, cosmic view includes *'order in the chaos.'* And when you include soul contracts, lessons learned and the contrasts we have set up in our game of life that is governed by the Spiritual and natural Laws of energy – we can safely conclude that – no matter what it is – "It's all good!" Learning lessons by painful experience can be very effective! However, the sooner we learn how to play the game energetically the way it works and clearly see what is going on, the less we have to repeat the painful patterns in our lives that don't work.

All boats lead to China, even the slow boats. But as far as 'getting there' is concerned, most 'rowers' agree that having a *motor* on the boat is better than having to use *oars for such a long distance.* And that having a computer *processor* that runs *fast* and is reliable is better than having one that runs *slow* and is *unreliable* for clearly processing information.

So what this really means is that our problems come from our inability to sufficiently ascertain and process what our problems really are, and then perform their solutions clearly, quickly and appropriately with positive consistency to regenerate our life, body, businesses and relationships. And how can we do this unless we know how the game of energy that we all must play is set up?

Einstein said, "God doesn't play dice with the Universe" – meaning there is *order in the Universe.* Reality is defined by the Laws of energy in the sciences of physics and metaphysics. Without order, it would be like playing basketball where everybody makes up their own rules as they go along!

Such a game would not *look* like basketball because there would be *no order* to define the game so the energy of all those in the game would be forced to fight over whose rules will rule! By definition, such a game *would not even begin to look like basketball.* Also, it would be impossible to win such a game since nobody would agree upon any common 'Reality' of rules to define what is, and what is not 'Real.'

In our personal energy game of life, the Rules are the Laws of energy, and energy always operates according to the Laws of energy. These Laws, natural Laws of energy, are being played out everywhere all the time – just like the energies of the stars and black holes, which operate in the Universe in perfect order that aligns with the Laws of energy.

To win our game of life (or any game) we must first learn the Rules and know how to use our Tools to align with the *Ways, Rules and Laws* so 'the force' of the Laws of Life-force energy is *with us* (to regenerate and give us personal power) – rather than being unconsciously directed *against us* (as drag that creates disease, disorder, dysfunction and degeneration).

Consciously knowing and conceptually understanding how we function energetically as a whole *integrated organic system* (validated by infrared science) clarifies how we are designed to function to regenerate. We can do this by consciously getting ahead of our triggered reactive drag on our Life-force energy so it flows naturally from what we *see* and *feel* to what we *think, say and do.*

When we feel safe and worthy of love as children, then our energy flows naturally and follows these Ways of Spirit and Laws of energy unconsciously. Our 'processing time' is instant and spontaneous. This changes if we are *traumatized* and become self-conscious from experiencing *fear* of being true to our Self or Who we are. The un-traumatized child is one who has a *knowing* that is free of resistance to Truth.

Our more conscious children today are becoming more pure and connected to themselves. There is evidence that suggests the 'new kids,' the 'indigo' children, the 'star seeds,' the 'crystal' and 'rainbow' children, all seem to have a clearer idea of *Who they are.* In spite of the fact that many of them have parents who do not 'see,' these children often see with simple clarity.

These new children with their new clarity do seem to be more willing to take on old, authoritarian systems that no longer work. In fact, they seem more willing to do things differently, in ways that make more sense. Most of them are even blessed with great gifts of artistry, music and clairvoyant abilities as well so that the entire world can be consciously upgraded just for having them in it. Their light here shows us the many ways Spirit Life-force energy can manifest when it is 'online' and working in the human vehicle!

Processing Life at the Speed of Light

Clairvoyance is the ability to intuitively and spontaneously 'do the math' on what aligns with the Laws of energy so we can see the results of those Laws in our mind's eye almost instantly as to how different decisions will play out in real time. As we become more capable of such consistent clarity in our consciousness, we become much more secure and connected to our own deep inner knowing so we can operate from a centered new level of *clarified functioning* in our personal and collective consciousness.

This clarity and consciousness is becoming more available to us now as our planet and our entire solar system enters a new energy field of light above the horizontal galactic plane (photon belt) of our Milky Way Galaxy into the northern hemisphere where our solar system has not been in over 13,000 years. Mayan, religious, and astrological prophesies (and many other ancient cultural philosophies) all point to *this period of time* as marking the beginning of the *'Golden Age of Enlightenment.'* This is when humanity enters a whole different galactic polarity field of energy that enhances our ability to enlighten our conscious evolvement to better adapt to energetic Reality by *quickening* our ability to be more real.

And at a certain point in this transition, we will likely experience a *critical mass* of shifting consciousness to where the Light of Truth becomes the self-evident Way for many, if not for most everyone, to more clearly walk our path to fulfill our Spirit. This quantum evolutionary leap in consciousness will supposedly allow humans to become much more capable of processing an expanded subtle energy Reality, with much more consciousness connected to clarity. This will allow us to act more clearly and quickly in Ways that regenerate our Spirit's Life-force.

This shifting point of critical mass happens when we reach that point where a sufficient number of us align with the clarity of the Light of Truth to function consciously in our thoughts and actions. Many New Age writers have suggested this leap in human consciousness began to occur in 2012. We are indeed beginning to see and feel radical shifts and changes from reviewing and revaluing what is real in life and how to align with this human evolution going on all over the planet right now!

Knowing *Who we really are energetically* is essential for Spirit-driven people – who truly want to know what's real and act upon what they know. These are also the people most inclined to do their own personal consciousness work to be clearer and quicker in their decisions and actions directing their life.

To work on our personal consciousness, we must first have *a strong Spirit that is disciplined enough* to stay focused and aligned with energetic Reality. We must be willing to *see things clearly as they really are, and to see as we may have never seen before.* (This can be a humbling experience.)

Knowledge is power, so eventually this all boils down to the fact that when we do our consciousness work we become more filled with the Light of self-evident Truth so we more clearly and quickly perceive energetic Reality.

As we learn to more clearly perceive and express each organ/gland emotional energy function, we also learn better ways to express and communicate our 'organ/gland truths' more clearly, quickly and appropriately. This is the essence of being more effective and efficient in our processing of our life, going from identifying the *real cause* of our problems to creating the *real solutions* to them. This is what being *'more intelligent' is all about.*

The road to enlightenment has been described in many ways, but in some form or another, it always boils down to clearer and quicker processing time. This is the time it takes to go from getting clarity about what's causing our problems to enacting the solutions that eliminate our problems.

In Egypt, the figure of a serpent was worn in a headdress to symbolize a person who had *overcome the (dragon) serpent within themselves.* The serpent signified wisdom and eternal life (because when the serpent sheds its' skin, it is 'young again'). The people who wore this headdress had effectively demonstrated their ability to *discipline their serpent* or dragon energy and had *kept it from running their lives.* In order to accomplish this, these persons had honed their ability to *favor their Spirit* as their guide for achieving consciousness in alignment with their divine Self.

In the same way, when we have disciplined our reactive dragons, we can then see clearly both from within and without. This is the game we must win if we are ever to evolve or refine ourselves by discerning and discriminating among the energies of our world more clearly and quickly.

All great formulas are centered on a *constant*, which ties everything else together in an order of understanding. The constant in our own personal world of energy is still the Laws of energy, which determine how we get all of our points and penalties in our game of life.

Our points in life are determined by *how well we perform* in alignment with the Rules and Laws of life's energy game. As I mentioned before, we're all forced to play this energy game, every day – even if we aren't consciously aware of how life's energy game works. And yet, this performance is what determines the outcome of *everything in our life*.

My observations come from working with thousands of clients over many years that have shown me how things change when they direct their actions with clearer and quicker decisions that are more connected to their truth and energetic Reality – which resolves many of their symptoms and problems on all the different levels of their personal functioning.

Our Point of Power

I once heard the Dalai Lama being asked, "Would you be willing to negotiate the conflicts of your Tibetan people, with the Chinese government?" He immediately responded, "Of course, if they will accept Reality." (Apparently, the Dalai Lama knew that there is *no point in negotiating with anyone who will not accept Reality!* Such clear quick processing is what we expect from the Dalai Lama's consciousness!)

The bottom line is this: If we don't align our decisions and actions with Reality so we can live in alignment with Reality – then we must expect the problems created from living misaligned with Reality!

When the messages from our problematic symptoms of degenerating mass are properly decoded, they reveal the elegant solutions to our problems. Seeing this consciously enables us to know and understand so we may have the choice to consciously change our unconscious decisions that are creating our problems – into more conscious decisions and actions that will create our elegant solutions.

My experience has been that this only happens if and when we clearly decode our symptomatic messages from the body's own language of our organ/gland energies and their Laws/Ways. Doing this reveals and enlightens our regenerative pathways with decisions in the present that create what we want in our future (versus making decisions in the present as if we were reliving our past – which recreates our past in our present!).

If we can process, live and direct our Life-Force energy with sufficient enlightened alignment with our truth guiding us, we will create 'enlightened alignment' with Reality so we may be able to sustain that alignment long enough to override the opposition of drag to manifest our Spirit's truth.

The power of enlightenment is being able to consciously respond clearly, quickly and appropriately to most any stimulus, spontaneously, within a second or less ¬¬to have power over our moments of truth! The reason our in-the-moment response is so important is because that moment is our moment of power – when our maximum potential personal power actually exists!

The importance of this Reality relating to our response time (inter-stimulus interval) is confirmed by learning research in psychology. This research shows that: "Conditioning is not noticeably affected by the schedule of reinforcement when the inter-stimulus interval is long, but is markedly influenced at the 1.1-second interval [when the inter-stimulus interval is short]." [*Foundations of Conditioning and Learning*, by Gregory A. Kimble; Appleton Century Crofts, 1967, p. 654]

This means we lose personal power in our daily life when we are not capable of being spontaneously clear and quick in our true perceptions, and able to appropriately express our truth – within slightly <u>over</u>

one second from any stimulus. This is what I am always referring to as our 'moment of truth,' because it is our moment of power.

It's a lot like training a dog. The ideal time interval between the *stimulus* (peeing on the carpet) and our *response* (communicating it's *not* ok), must consistently be near that 1.1 second interval (of the dog peeing on carpet) in order for optimal learning to occur. This is when our personal power to stop it peaks.

Otherwise, we operate in sub-optimal personal power as a dog trainer, because the dog finds us confusing and not believable, and if nobody believes us, we don't have any power. This self-evident example shows us how a *short interval* (between behavior and response) *is the most powerful consideration* for 'learning' to occur and it also *defines our ability to have personal power.*

Therefore, our *optimal 'point of personal power'* in any aspect of our life (business, social and personal relationships) comes down to our ability to clearly and appropriately respond to the stimulus within one second. In other words, it's all about being instantly clear and present with any challenge. If we can respond clearly, quickly and appropriately to the stimulus within that second, we will have maximum power for being most effective and productive at accomplishing whatever it is we want to accomplish.

Understanding and aligning our decisions and actions with the energetic Laws of Spirit and nature gives us guidelines for living in the grace of the Laws and Ways with personal respect for energetic Reality. This is the natural flow that aligns with the Laws of energy so 'The Force' of those Laws is with us (which gives us our personal power)! (The two 'forces' are the magnetic force of the dragon and the Life-force of our Spirit. When referring to Spirit Life-force in this book, we will capitalize 'The Force'.)

Our *quality of life* is determined by *how well we align* what we *see* and *feel* with what we *say* and *do*.

'The Force' that comes from this alignment regenerates us. Otherwise, if we *see* one thing, *feel* another thing, *say* another thing, and *do* another thing – we are, by definition, *disintegrating*. And if we do that long enough, our lives, bodies, businesses and relationships will *disintegrate*! (These four brain-lobe/memory functions are what the hippies were talking about when they said, "Get it together man" – get together what you are *seeing* and *feeling* together with what you are *saying* and *doing*.)

Our four cerebral lobes, or memory banks (of seeing, saying, feeling, and doing) are integrated parts that comprise 80% of our brain as four pairs of lobes comprising our cerebral cortex. They are: *occipital* (visual: seeing, space); *temporal* (mental: understanding, linear time); *kinesthetic* (emotional: feeling, experiences); and *motor* (physical: doing, moving and performing).

Carolyn Myss, the bestselling author of *Anatomy of the Spirit,* has an audiotape entitled *"Why People Don't Heal,"* where she says that the main reason people don't heal is because *healing is an act of creation.* This means that we must *create* our own healing, and to do so we must be consciously focused on and do what heals us at least **85%** of our time in order for us to be sufficiently engaged in conscious healing action enough for the Laws of creation to heal us. (Not doing so is what is creating our problems.)

This means that *if we are not continuously making decisions and taking actions that are creating our solutions,* then we are likely to be continuing to unconsciously make decisions and take actions that are creating our problems – *so they cannot ever go away!*

So, when we focus on our fears, we are actually creating more reasons to fear, because fear usually stops our ability to create solutions – since what you focus on is what you create. We are often unable to *connect with, act from and focus on* what we love, because we are way too focused on what we fear. And fear causes us to see from a place of confusion instead of the 'big picture window' of solutions.

Fear prevents us from healing because it prevents us from staying focused on what heals us long enough for healing to actually occur. In the meantime, confusion and disconnection create more confusion and disconnection – from thinking, acting and being in c*onfusion and disconnection.*

> ***Often 'the problem' is what perpetuates the problem that prevents the solution to the problem.***

When this happens it becomes a 'down and in' degenerative cycle of *unconscious* self-destruction and dysfunction that we pay for dearly. And because this degenerative cycle is so common it creates a real need for a *conscious* 'health care plan' that is firmly based in energetic

Reality. A conscious health care plan would be one that scientifically individualizes personal programming in relation to specific health problems.

Chapter 3

Science that Scans, Measures, and Tracks Drag on Energy Flow

What I Learned From My PhD

Early in my career, I had no science to measure and decode my clients' subtle-energy flow patterns to see how their problems were being unconsciously programmed by their trauma memory. Nor could I scientifically track their energy flow patterns over time and connect the dots for them about what organ/gland energies were degenerating – and why and where and how to regenerate them. And I certainly had no idea they needed to learn to consciously perceive and express their organ/gland energies clearly, quickly and appropriately in order to solve their problems.

After doing my doctoral training and dissertation research and then using biofeedback as my clinical scientific tool in therapy with clients I still felt I did not have what I needed to give my clients what they came to me to get. Still, after receiving my doctorate and practicing psychology for thirteen years (1974-1987), I came to realize that even after my PhD and using the best traditional scientific psychology had to offer (biofeedback at that time) for integrating and connecting the mind and body functionally and scientifically, I STILL could not clearly, quickly and scientifically identify and/or decode my clients' specific unconscious programming – which at this point I knew was the real root of their problems, even though I had no solution to that problem – yet.

So with all of my training, practice and clinical knowledge gleaned from my clients and extensive human research, I still had no way to quickly and easily get to the root of my clients' personal issues that were programming their problems! Yet I knew there had to be a way that it would be possible to decode our human programming in order to clearly show, scientifically, how humans work *energetically*.

Being unable to even begin to clarify what seemed essential to provide elegant fulfilling solutions for my clients' problems was the onset of my professional depression, and for good reason! In retrospect, I can see that I had no tools to scientifically clarify my clients' problems so I could effectively and efficiently direct them on how to enact the elegant solutions to their problems by functioning more consciously aligned with who they are.

I wanted to find a way to scientifically show how humans work energetically to be able to decode their individual programming into how they are unconsciously creating their personal problems. I figured that then it would be possible to help them raise their consciousness for how/when they are creating specific problems. Until this was accomplished, I realized that it would be impossible to assist my clients to learn to stop unconsciously creating their problems, and start consciously creating their elegant solutions.

Without the tools to do my job, I was frequently very unclear in my own understanding about how trauma memory actually programs how we think and process our feelings and what we see in our mind's eye. Without a human map it is hard to find our way around our energetic territory! And therefore I could not provide any of my clients with real, effective solutions to any of their human energetic problems, because I had still not figured it out myself.

Working with biofeedback helped me to see how closely correlated physical responses were to more subtle, energetic stimuli. And I was convinced that our spiritual, mental, emotional and physical bodies could all 'talk' to one another. The questions were: "If that were true, then what exactly are they saying to each other?" And: "How were they doing it?"

I had a breakthrough of sorts one day when I realized that the *issues are in the tissues.* This seemed to be the key to everything if my premise was correct that there was a true correlation between all the systems in a perfected design. And since the *issues are in the tissues,* there must be a way to scientifically integrate and understand the entire human system. But, without adequate scientific tools or sufficiently clear organic concepts for how humans function as a whole integrated energy system, I realized that I could never have or provide a clear understanding of what actually happens with an individual client energetically between their mind, body, emotions and Spirit Life-force energy that will either create their disease – or their fulfillment.

Over many years, listening to so many people's troubles, I realized that all human problems come down to being unconsciously and instantly triggered into time-warped re-lives of specific defensive decisions and actions. These, over time, manifest as denser and denser energy problems – manifesting as disease, disorder, dysfunction, and degeneration – that evolve from being issues in our life to showing up in the tissues of our body.

Then I realized these problems are only resolved when we become sufficiently conscious to see and get ahead of our triggered unconscious decisions in our moments of power so we can replace our decisions that are creating our problems – with new decisions that will create our solutions. It is a *dance of energy* within us. I was constantly repeating that 'it was all about energy.'

And even though I was always saying that it was 'all about energy,' it still became more and more clear to me that it is nearly impossible to fix anything while still laboring in confusion. I needed clarity about what our tools are and how to use them to facilitate regenerative ways that create our solutions and avoid creating our problems! (The Hippocratic oath gives us the first axiom of healing which is: "First, do no harm." And without a fully integrative healing method, what else could be the end result when we are never getting to the actual root of any given problem?)

Eventually, my research and discoveries led to a realization that all humans first need to be able to consciously overwrite our reactive unconscious memory of dysfunctional decisions by scripting and practicing new functional behavior patterns – instead of repeating our past memories (of dysfunctional patterns) that are creating our problems. Then I could see that we must also be able to express specific organ/ gland energies clearly, quickly and appropriately.

After I could clearly see and conceptually understanding exactly how we program our problems and our solutions – I could also see how critically essential that insight is for all clients to know for their own health. Only then could I feel I could give them what they need to become conscious enough of their own energetic Reality to get ahead of their reactivity to walk an enlightened path in their moments of truth.

I realized what every Spirit wants concerning every problem is first energetic clarity concerning their problem, so they can see exactly how they are creating and maintaining their problems. Then they can begin operate ahead of the curve to make clearer decisions quicker followed by effective actions to create their elegant solution and prevent their problem as soon as possible.

I also had to realize that no dragon (trauma memory) is ever interested in enlightening plans about energetic Reality because this energy is only capable of defensive solutions using the 'dragon's ways' to endure and survive without solutions by using deception to manipulate the confused with fear and force!

What I learned is that all Spirits need a conscious clear, simple energetic view of who we are and how we function energetically to see and figure out the elegant solutions to our problems. I knew that if I could get a basic clear, scientific perception of who we all are and how we all function energetically as humans, I would then have a firm baseline foundation on which to build a true scientific picture of how each individual is integrated to personally function energetically in terms of their own programming.

In order to do this I needed an energetic scientific tool that would track and reveal our *organic codes* that connect the dots of our *energetic flow patterns* and show how our specific *life* issues relate to our decisions and actions that associate with specific memory and degenerative *organ/gland issues/tissues.*

I needed to be able to link measured electrical energy flow patterns (energy-motion codes) from trauma memory with how we make unconscious decisions that program our organ/gland emotional dysfunctions and physical degeneration that age us.

I have found this level of energetic clarity about organ/gland energy functions is critically essential to empower motivated people by giving them sufficient consciousness to create their elegant solutions that prevent and *avoid* their degenerative problems.

I have also found that elegant solutions first require perceiving clearly and then expressing the right dose at the right time – to give us sufficient power to claim our life and maintain our personal power. But before all these breakthroughs, my own personal power in my profession was at a standstill. And at this time in my life, I didn't know which direction to go.

My Dad always told me that in order to do a job well, you had to have the right tools. In fact, I was so frustrated, that even after working hard for 20 years to get my PhD, and working nonstop for 13 years in my chosen field, I thought about quitting all the time. I didn't really want to, but I could see where the end of the road was, and I could see that it wasn't what I had 'signed up for.' I was at a crossroads and I knew it. What was next for me? If anyone knew – I was wishing they would tell me as I pondered the several roads in front of me.

I was still excited about the 'fully integrated medicine' idea, but the body had not yet unlocked all its' emotional secrets to me. And behind those locks was a writhing humanity in pain and frustration while at the same time poised on the edge of enlightenment. Just like me.

It was a hard time for me, but this is when I learned how dead ends can be expanding experiences if you can see clearly and stay open to future possibilities. But still – nothing could have prepared me for what I was about to run into next in the way of 'mind blowing expansion' in a highly specialized field of learning! And looking back, I can't see this as anything but a well laid out plan for two researchers in the exact same field to meet.

Infrared Science Shows Human Functioning as an Integrated Whole

Finally, I became so frustrated with my inadequate psychological tools (including biofeedback) that I gave up my entire practice of psychology and began working in a totally different profession! However, as fate would have it, within a few months of my leaving psychology, in 1987 I met Joseph R. Scogna, who was using infrared science to discover, track and map integrated human organ/gland energetic functioning!

This experience changed me quickly and dramatically because I had a chance to see with my own eyes the basics of how true integrative science works!

This occurred during that first evening when I met Joseph Scogna and he did his infrared scan on my girlfriend Arlene after she had just spent most of that day scrubbing an unventilated bathroom with ammonia. Without having had any previous conversation with Arlene, and never having seen her before, Joe looked at her chain of numbers from her scan and asked, "How did you get toxic poisoning from ammonia?"

This incredibly surprising and powerful revelation shocked me and instantly changed my life and career back into psychology as

a measurable integrated science of consciousness! Because I knew immediately that in order to decode that specific information (ammonia poisoning) from Arlene's infrared measurement, Joe had to have connected a lot of scientific dots in-between. And that's what I had been looking for – for many, many years at that point!

I soon learned that the most significant 'dots in-between' were all of the organ/gland emotional (energy-motion) issues that provide immense clinical value! In fact, they make it possible to decode/decipher insights from subtle organ/gland functioning, in less than a minute, from a total stranger – without ever having even to touch or talk to the person!

I was also soon to discover that the emotional issues that parallel specific organ/glands tissues with problems were even more stunning in terms of how they provided personal insights into the effects of trauma memory programming, and how the clearer our energetic view is of who we are and how we function, the more possibilities we have for being conscious as Spirit Life-force Beings in a human body!

Finally, I had the science I had dreamed of since my doctoral dissertation research and from then on, I felt like I was light years ahead of my old biofeedback view of human energetic Reality!

It was profound for me to have a tool that scientifically reveals a mirror-image energetic view of our personal energetic programming in an organic (organ/gland) language that integrates physical functioning with our *emotional* processing and *mental* (including trauma memory) programming of our Spirit Life-force organ/gland energy.

This work provided insights about humans that changed my life forever. I learned about using infrared science to reveal the 'organic energy maps' for how we program our organ/gland Spirit Life-force (mental-emotional-physical) energy flow circuits. By measuring and tracking our energy flow circuits over time, our coded disease patterns reveal their connections to our unconsciously associated trauma memory, which then programs our decisions and actions that create most of our problems.

These energy flow patterns reveal the secrets to our personal powers and problems by revealing our *natural organ/gland language,* which runs our system from conception. This happens when our twenty-three pairs of mother/father chromosomes connect to form the nucleus of our original cell at conception. Then we develop through a 280-day process of gestation, from conception to the birth of our body (with twenty-three integrated Spirit Life-force organ/gland mental/ emotional/physical systems and functions).

Infrared measurements of the energy flow patterns between these organ/gland energy systems track and reveal mirror-image levels of physical/emotional/mental energy functioning (and dysfunctioning) that specifically detail individual 'blocked circuit' problems and their solutions, that are revealed in our innate organic language of twenty-three organ/gland energy systems. Our *organic language* of 'degenerative order' was first revealed in studies about the effects of radiation on the human body. When humans are exposed to intense radiation (or less intense consistent stress over sufficient time), our organs/glands degenerate and age in a very specific and particular order, according to their importance for survival. When we combine the 'organic language' (from the radiation studies) with 'infrared science', we get a *personalized and integrated science of Life-force energy* that provides our own personal energetic map.

This map organically decodes the unconscious source of our defensive decisions (trauma memory) that are blocking specific Life-force energies with 'drag' that is *degenerating* us. And the map also reveals how and what is needed to *regenerate* these powers. It is also the *perfect consciousness tool,* enabling us to connect the energetic 'dots' of personal insights with consciousness sufficient to be clear enough quickly enough to make choices that prevent and change our dysfunctional problems into our functional regenerative solutions.

Once I started using infrared science with an organic format to decode all my clients, I really learned how our natural organic language works. I was then able to measure, track and decode personal energy flow patterns that revealed deep secrets about how these patterns relate to programming their health and disease. The nature of our energetic language is like a *Rosetta stone* – which turns gibberish into clarity.

By using an organic format we get organic insights that allow us to see our different mirror image levels of organ/gland energy functions. These functions integrate to tell us the specific unconscious decisions and actions that are creating our problems (from the natural energetic effects of the Laws of energy), as well as the conscious decisions and actions that will create *solutions* to those specific problems!

In sum, our mental thoughts and emotional memory are designed to program and direct our Spirit's Life-force energy through our emotional feeling experiences as either expressing them to hopefully create solutions, or suppressing them to eventually create emotional and physical effects or emotional problems.

Our organ/gland language decodes, integrates and explains how all our levels of mental, emotional and physical energy function together to create all the problems and solutions in our life and body!

Our organic language consists of twenty-three organ/gland energy systems that flow through 253 Life-force energy circuits and reveal unique individual patterns of drag. These flow patterns of drag can be measured and tracked by infrared and organically decoded to reveal our unconscious programming for meaningful energetic insights that allow us to consciously getting ahead of old, familiar, unconscious, dysfunctional decision patterns directing our life from old, reactive habits.

With the clarity of infrared science integrated around an organic organ/gland format, I finally had hope for a real integrated science of human health, with a clear detailed view of organ/gland energy degeneration. I finally had a real energetic science that *measured, tracked and revealed* how our mental and emotional programming integrates to function energetically with the precision of mathematics!

I have always considered this science most worthy of my time, energy and focus because it reveals an energetic mirror-image that is a map of all our Life-force energy flow, which reveals our systems' emotional trauma programming that is creating our problems energetically!

Since that day when I saw what was revealed from Arlene's scan, I have not focused on anything else. Now I have a clear, simple organic decoding tool that works for every human. This reality has exceeded my scientific expectations far beyond my wildest dreams of possibilities that I could have ever imagined! It finally scientifically integrates psychology, biology and physics and is what I have come to refer to as: **'psycho-bio-physics.'**

This is a clinically proven valid scientific tool that I have used for twenty-five years to measure, track, decode and translate subtle energy flow patterns into personal symptomatic messages to reveal unconscious decision patterns that are creating my clients problems, so together we can facilitate changing their decisions and actions to create their solutions.

Now we use the insights from my client's 'infrared programming code' (a numerical chain) to clearly show how the decisions they are making in their life connects to their body problems and how they are maintaining those patterns daily in their actions or performances. Seeing the individual scenes (good and bad) *clearly* in the movie of their life allows them to raise their personal consciousness by finally *seeing what their life looks like* as a movie in terms of how it works to attract or repel audiences or create what you want. It's all in the 'movie of their life.'

We do this by providing expanded concepts based on science that allow us to see and understand how and why we must perform what our solution messages are telling (from their infrared scan) that they need to do in order to achieve what their Spirit wants. We carefully study what each specific organ/gland energy pattern is revealing from their infrared measurements, so that the client can perceive and express him or herself in a way that achieves the desired life changes to create fulfillment.

My experience has taught me how to clearly and effectively read, interpret and communicate about the subtle energy realms so people can become more conscious of their unconscious behavior. With *The BodyTalker Emotional Infrared Science* I now do all of this with every client. The process is simple, yet the information obtained is profound and amazingly accurate, consistent and naturally integrated.

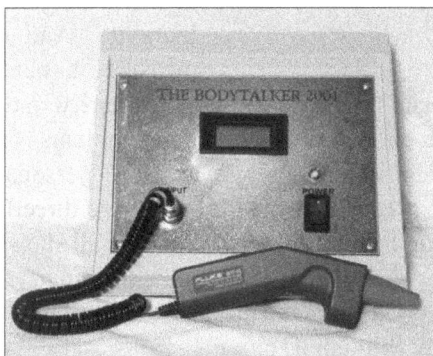

*Shown above is the 2001 version of **The BodyTalker** emotional infrared scanning system that takes measurements from our face vector/ junction points that are shown in the illustration below.*

The BodyTalker infrared science reads the body's electrical energy flow patterns (between our twenty-three organ and glands) by scanning these junction points on the face. The scan reveals blocked energy flow patterns between specific organs and glands, which correspond to specific physiological symptoms, emotional dysfunctions and mental confusions that are directing the client's decisions – that are directing their lives

The Face Matrix Junction Points and Their Circuits of Power

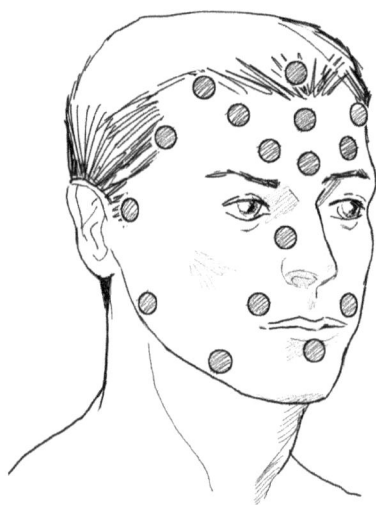

The illustration here shows our Life-force energy vector/junction points. Our Life-force energy flows through these points, to and from our organs and glands to give us the power and energy to perceive and perform all of our physical, emotional and mental Spirit Life-force energy functions. Everyone talks about personal power, but unless you are familiar with this science, nobody is quantifying it, integrating it and individualizing it. And unless you can measure it, personalize it, and translate it, you can't be very helpful to clarify and assist them to become conscious enough to change their problems.

In other words, as humans, we have 253 personal powers which are related to our organs and glands which are directly related to our problems when our circuits are blocked. This all shows up as a matrix of energy that can 'speak' to us if we know the language it is speaking! It is a language that all humans are designed to understand since it is about 253 two way (binomial) circuits.

Speaking scientifically, the face matrix force vector junction points map out our 253 Life-force energy circuits of our powers to perform the 253 permutations (all the different combinations) of our twenty-three Organ/Gland Energy systems (which represent our 253 powers and problems). When we see ourselves this way, energetically – we are really a very simple system that boils down to 253 potential blocked circuits or 253 flowing circuits – depending on how conscious we are of our system and what is decisions we make that are regenerative or degenerative.

The blocked circuits (of trauma memory) show up on infrared to reveal how a person is creating their problems as well as how to create their solutions. The organ/gland language combined with the infrared science provides a massive amount of integrated health information showing how mental, emotional, and physical issues all interrelate.

Below is an example of only the first issue – (which is safety) for the first organ – the thymus (represented by the number 1). Each of the numbers indicates a specific organ/gland and its issues that are associated with the thymus (1-2 = thymus and heart, 1-3 = thymus and colon, etc). This is what we call an uplink and these are examples of what an uplink means and how it shows up from the infrared read out. It is a blocked circuit between two specific organs and glands. Below we are showing the first set of 22 uplinks out of 253 circuits so you can see how the human system works energetically.

1 – 2. Safety and Love = Feeling safe and worthy of love

1 – 3. Safety and Hate = Feeling safe to eliminate what we hate

1 – 4. Safety and Happiness = Feeling safe to choose what makes us happy

1 – 5. Safety and Control = Feeling safe to master, control and direct our life

1 – 6. Safety and Transmutation = Feeling safe to transmute what we've got into what we want

1 – 7. Safety and Breathing = Feeling safe to breath into our challenges

1 – 8. Safety and Connection = Feeling safe to open up and connect with others

1 – 9. Safety and Movement = Feeling safe to approach/avoid what we want/don't want

1 – 10. Safety and Justice = Feeling safe taking action to correct what's not right

1 – 11. Safety and Circulation = Feeling safe to participate in the games of life

1 – 12. Safety and Simplicity = Feeling safe to simplify our lives by being true to our Self

1 – 13. Safety and Courage = Feeling safe to meet pressure with equal and opposite pressure

1 – 14. Safety and Wonder = Feeling safe to wonder and create how things could be

1 – 15. Safety and Communication = Feeling safe to perceive and communicate our truth

1 – 16. Safety and Filtering = Feeling safe to filter what does not work for us

1 – 17/18. Safety and Survival = Feeling safe to do what is necessary to survive

1 – 19. Safety and Identity = Feeling safe to define and defend our true identity

1 – 20. Safety and Expression = Feeling safe to express our true feelings

1 – 21. Safety and Grief = Feeling safe to grieve and process feelings of loss

1 – 22. Safety and Anger = Feeling safe to decisively say what we really want/don't want

1 – 23. Safety and Antagonism = Feeling safe to reject what disrespects us

1 – 24. Safety and Clarity = Feeling safe to be clear and accept only what regenerates us

Confused decisions (relating to the above circuits for example) manifest into our body, business and relationship problems that will eventually manifest as disease, disorder and dysfunction messages. *If* our unconsciously programmed decisions don't become conscious so we know where, when, how and what dysfunctional decisions and actions we are making when (or before) we are making them, then we are not conscious enough, in our moments of power, to re-script our lines and express them effectively enough to create the results our Spirit desires. This all relates to knowing where our blocked circuits are located as well as what those locations mean in reference to the specific issues we are having – which is why infrared coupled with the organic language of the body is so revealing.

Remember, showing up in our personal moments-of-power allows us to be believable by just being real, clear and spontaneously appropriate (within 1.1 sec following the stimulus) so we are effective in our 'moments of truth.' This is when we have the most learning influence or personal power, if we respond appropriately by making decisions that regenerate us instead of degenerate our energy. If we know where our blocked circuits are, we can have a heightened awareness for when/where and how our human problems are manifesting as confusions (decisions and actions) in our moments of power (which is when most decisions are made that direct our life and body).

It has not been easy for science to clearly perceive, theorize, hypothesize, measure, track, analyze and explain how the subtle energies of trauma memory reactively program our Spirit Life-force energy to degenerate from defensive unconscious decisions made reactively.

Other medical technologies also use infrared science to display visual infrared images that they use as their data for interpretations. Some others use electromagnetic frequencies of various energies in and of the body to view disease energy.

However, simply seeing these blocks in the body that comes from our trauma memory programming of drag on our Spirit Life-force energy flow does not provide us with anything close to what is essential to create real elegant integrated solutions to our problems!

> *No pictures or frequencies of our energy blocks and problems will ever be able to decode our unconsciously programmed 'drag' on our Spirit Life-force energy 'flow' (between our organs/glands) that creates our health and energy problems!*

The BodyTalker uses infrared science to gather data (the density of electrons) by measuring specific 'force vector' points on the human face that are the 'junction points' for the flow of electrical energy between each of the twenty-three organ/gland energy systems. This method of using infrared to measure scientifically how Life-force energy flows or drags through all our binomial circuits of power is a significant advantage over using visual pictures or frequencies to identify, translate and decode our health problems.

In summary, as humans we are all 253 circuits of potential energy that is flowing, partially flowing, or blocked. Optimally, our electrical energy is designed to flow (input/output) through our 253 binomial (two-way) circuits of power, which provides our basic 253 personal powers. When we learn to allow our powers of perception and expression to flow clearly, quickly and appropriately (with a real smile that shows a loving intent with a quest for the truth and a great sense of humor), this allows us to not take things too personally or seriously. Doing this well allows us to create just about *anything* our Spirit desires, by giving the time it takes to learn to do what creates what we want, and then just focusing on doing what is required to create it.

Consciousness: Our Future's Most Essential Survival Skill

A *science of consciousness* is essential in order to map and decode human energy flow patterns to reveal our problems and resolve our solutions by first becoming conscious of our unconscious decisions that are creating most of our human functioning problems. These problems usually stem from not perceiving Reality clearly and expressing our truth effectively enough to manifest our Spirit's desires and solutions.

Since 1987 I have been using the body's own natural 'organic language' to track and decode my clients' electrical energy flow patterns in order to shine light on their unconsciously programmed decisions that are creating their problems and preventing their elegant solutions.

Having had the ability to scientifically observe thousands of client energy flow patterns for over twenty-five years, I've seen more and more clearly how our emotional and mental 'dots' connect to how we are programmed to create our emotional dysfunctions and physical diseases. This has allowed me to see 'up close and personal' how the human system develops. Knowing this often reveals what our problems are years before they would ever show up as physical diseases!

Energy flow patterns are now almost a foreign concept in healthcare – but once the integrated language of our body's organs and glands are clearly understood, I am sure that energy flow patterns will be included in future health consideration!

Having conscious conceptual insight for how life's energy game happens gives us the power to perform 'ahead of the curve' in our moments of power. When this is perfected to where we live in this conscious space continuously, we will then be living in and leading healthy, regenerative and fulfilling lives.

No matter how we analyze human problems, the underlying aspect is always how they exist energetically. Elegant solutions, when seen clearly, always reveal themselves as being *self-evident and undeniable facts of energetic Reality*. Whenever anything energetically can be consciously conceptualized quickly to create a clear map of the energetic territory, then we are much more able to make conscious, effective and productive decisions and actions from our clarity for how things are before they happen.

Some New Age writers claim we are currently experiencing a 'quickening' time period, when humans are being forced by the Universe to become *clearer more quickly* about energetic Reality just to keep up with and solve the ever increasing stuff we must *process* to live life. Now begins the Age of 'Knowing,' the keynote of the new Age of Aquarius! We are now leaving the Age of 'believing' (Pisces) after 2000 years of believing in *One* who Knows (Jesus, Buddha, et. al.), and are now reaching that stage of consciously knowing energetic Reality instead of just believing in 'One' who Knows energetic Reality.

This transition from believing in 'isms' (about whatever one can imagine) – to Knowing God's Laws of physics (Reality as it actually exists energetically) and then following the Laws of subtle energy physics that align with our Spirit Ways – is a major transitional challenge in developing personal consciousness!

We currently face the inevitable challenge of dramatic change into a more subtle and refined dimension of energetic Reality. As we live through this evolutionary transition we are being forced to process more *input* clearer and quicker from our perceptions and then be able to express it more consciously in our *output*, by acting with more speed and clarity. We are going to have to do this just to stay even with our currently accelerating and evolving experience of transiting into a new dimension of energetic Reality!

Consciousness is consequently rapidly becoming *our most essential survival skill* for living effectively and productively in the twenty-first century!

Our current period is one of massive changes. We are living in an unconscious world where power and control keeps us confused and manipulated by the dragon's ways of deception, fear and force. But soon we will evolve into living consciously in a world that is not based on fear, but rather is becoming ordered around Love and Light, and aligned with the ethics of clear conscious performances of our Spirit's truth that increases our effectiveness, efficiency and productivity.

Our new world global economy will mirror the manifestations of these new views of Truth. And more and more, all Spirits will endeavor to work together to solve our own personal and global problems. As we consciously stay ahead of unconscious interference from triggered dragon memories, we can stay on the 'clearer, quicker path' always staying ahead of 'the reactive curve' in order to enable, inspire and maintain our Spirit's elegant solutions.

Otherwise, our lack of consciousness will result in dysfunctional reactive decisions in the moment that will lead us into fear-directed reactions that disconnect us from our centered empowered solutions from Source. And we must stay connected with and follow our Spirit's truth to fulfill and regenerate us.

Scientific energetic *tools* of consciousness help shine light on our personal energetic pathways. These enlighten and clarify our subtle energy realms of unconscious programming for who we are and how we function through our twenty-three Spirit Life-force organ/gland energies.

Infrared subtle energy technology enables us to measure, track, translate and explain, using energetic concepts that bring to light a much bigger, clearer, verifiable picture of who we are and how we function.

Each of our twenty-three organ/gland systems is designed to perceive and express their Life-force energy through each of their binomial two-way connections between each of our twenty-three organ/gland energy systems. This is done through 253 circuits of electrical energy flowing through our body with our own Life-force energy.

These streams of Life-force energy that flow through our electrical energy circuits can be measured with infrared science. This breaks new ground in the field of subtle energy science that integrates physical, emotional and mental programming of our health and illness.

Perhaps the bigger picture is about how our system is programmed to maintain 'homeostasis by drag' if and when it does not have the ability to make more conscious choices to make clearer quicker decisions and take more effective actions that prevent and eliminate our problems and create real sustainable solutions. (This is the reason consciousness is the only elegant solution to human problems.)

Genetic scientists call 97% of our DNA "junk DNA," apparently because they don't know what it does. But do you really think God created the 97% of our DNA to be junk? And if the 97% of our DNA (that is beyond the protein level) is not junk, we must be just barely at the beginning of making much more enlightened discoveries about how our consciousness relates to our health.

By doing a 'Reality check' on the consciousness of our current *views* and *behaviors*, we can begin to see and incorporate our own personal 'ah ha' insights (revealed when we decode our energy flow patterns) into new scripts and performances that can prevent our problems and create our solutions!

Only clarity and consciousness allow us to be clear enough and quick enough to override unconscious decisions that are creating our problems and preventing our solutions. This is how we avoid re-creating our old problems into new ones, and instead begin making decisions and actions that create our solutions.

Without the ability to measure, track and decode our refined unconscious subtle energy programming, elegant solutions are not easy to see and are often much less therapeutically possible. This is because of the major confusions caused by insufficient clarity about our uniquely personal and individual subtle energy memory and programming of our own experiences.

Now infrared scanning gives us the ability to energetically define and decode how humans are naturally integrated as individualized systems of Spirit Life-force energy with specific plans, issues, functions and traumas. Our Spirit Life-force energy is mostly programmed by a combination of clear conscious mental thinking and confused unconscious emotional memory of trauma that often shows up in our performance as hesitation. This 'drag' on our performance in our moments of power will also eventually show up in our body as physical symptoms – which are messages telling us what the solution is! This human design is already naturally built into your system!

Using infrared data the way the BodyTalker uses it to *track* and *decode* electrical flow patterns is a major advancement in understanding and enhancing human health. It enables us to observe where energy is blocked and where it is flowing and the ability to decode why these blocks are occurring in terms of the decisions being made that are creating these blocks in the body's Life-force energy currents. These infrared scans not only show blocked organ/gland circuits, but also reveal the blocked organ/gland functions plus the emotional issue and mental thinking that are creating it, as well as how to correct it. This gives us a very scientifically integrated conceptual view and understanding of our personal mental, emotional and physical organ/gland energy functions – and how they work as a whole integrated system.

Our Trauma-Fear-Resistance-Heat-Degeneration Disease Patterns

In its simplest form, trauma creates fear, causing resistance (or 'drag' on the flow of Life-force energy) that results in heat and degenerates tissues to create various diseases. So our issues of life that 'don't work' create resistance (heat) in the tissues of our body. This causes them to degenerate and eventually they become dysfunctional, cold and numb.

Our Spirit Life-force energy flows through various matrices of 'force-vector' points (energy flow junction points) throughout our body. These points serve to connect all of our organ/gland energy flow through circuitry that integrates our entire system of Life-force energy that gives us all our personal powers.

> *Twenty-first century tools must be able to measure refined human subtle-energy flow patterns, and decode them into clear messages quick enough to avoid problems and create solutions.*

Expression of our emotional feeling energy (energy-motion, or e-motion) is part of how we express our Spirit Life-force energy in an attempt to fulfill our divine intent by just being and expressing who we truly are – *without drag* on our truth and on Who we really are as Spirit Life-force energy of Love and Light!

Allowing our Spirit to consistently express who we truly are clearly, quickly and appropriately helps prevent all basic energetic problems in life – in health, business and relationships. This is because clear, quick and appropriate energetic perceptions and expressions regenerate and rejuvenate our entire Life-force energy system.

Once we've measured a person's infrared 'energy flow patterns' we can then decode their 'pattern/chain' to see how they are unconsciously programming their specific mental and emotional decisions that are creating their life, body, business and relationship problems.

We need *consciousness about energetic Reality* to become quick enough to override 'triggered' old familiar 'decision patterns' with decisions that prevent our problems and at the same time create regenerative and sustainable solutions for our life and body.

Analogous to a personal computer, our entire *human system is a bio-computer programmed by memory!* And we cannot effectively operate (or fix) our computer unless we understand how it works, know its operating system's 'language,' and how to use that language to function more freely with *more options quicker and with fewer problems!*

Now, by measuring, decoding and understanding our emotional (energy-motion) functioning with scientific clarity that reveals our deep personal programming, we can begin to see and operate from much clearer insights that direct a straighter path for expressing our truth and Who we really are, as a Spirit living in a material body!

Infrared Reveals Subtle 'Energy Flow Patterns'

Perfect solutions require perfectly clear observation
of the problem to be able to enact the elegant solution
that eliminates what is causing the problem.

Treating our physical effects is an impossibility until we understand more about how they are developed in the 'here and now' from the 'there and then.' First, we need to understand the fourth-dimensional source of our problems as being *memories of time. This is* a triggered memory of 'a time' (the fourth dimension is 'time') that creates a 'time-warp' in our moments of power, where a past reality is being unconsciously projected into our present reality. Without sufficient consciousness to operate from a *higher-dimensional subtle-energy view,* we cannot function on a continuous regenerative level of being! We cannot solve our Spirit-level human problems by treating them from a third-dimensional view (height-width-depth) of reality. In fact, *treating third-dimensional effects* is a futile effort that often adds to the long-term problem itself. Many of these treatments are dysfunctional and expensive but are still recommended by some traditional healthcare professionals.

In reality, our current 'health care system' is only 'emergency care' focused on *treating symptomatic effects* rather than the underlying *subtle energy causes* of confusion that create it. The confusion itself ensures that we could never become conscious enough to eliminate the cause of our problem – so we could stop creating our own problems. *This personal disempowerment is the root cause of a confused system from within as well as without.*

Now, by using infrared to scan and track our emotional energy flow patterns, we can scientifically and organically decode our subtle Spirit Life-force energy flow patterns programmed from trauma memory. This allows us to become conscious of (to get ahead of) our triggered, unconscious fourth-dimensional memory associations from making 'time-warped' projections of past decisions into our present decisions, which recreate our past problems in our present – by reliving them in our present. (This is the very essence of 'backward, defensive programming.')

Scientifically measuring, tracking and decoding our subtle-energy programming 'causes' – provides us with a much bigger, clearer picture of our personal energetic Reality than any dense matter observation of physical blocks ever could.

Our chances of accurately clearing our programmed issues are vastly increased when we have a way to measure, track and become consciously aware of how and when we are making specific decisions and actions (energy flow patterns) that create our dysfunctional effects (problems and diseases) so we can correct them.

When we can clearly see and consciously understand how our organ/gland energy system works – and know the energetic language of our operating system – we can now really have the choice to change our decisions and actions from creating our problems to creating our solutions by consciously overriding specific, unconscious decisions. If we do not energetically clear reactive 'dragon' memory with the light of consciousness, the emotional 'drag' of the issues creates an electrical 'drag' on Spirit Life-force energy flow which manifests in physical tissues.

It is our habits of re-enacting trauma memory that create and maintain our problems unconsciously. *Only* by being conscious enough to get ahead of them in or before our moments of decision can we decide to not do what we have always done. This means in order to prevent our problems from developing or continuing, we must learn to express our truth clearer, quicker and more appropriately.

The bottom line is that Real solutions inspire, regenerate and rejuvenate us, from expressing our true Spirit Life-force energy with actions that solve our problems with regenerative and sustainable solutions.

KNOW THYSELF

Chapter 4

Acknowledging Current "Health Care" Limitations

The Real Costs of Traditional Health Care

Traditional physiologically-based health care most often has inadequate and incomplete clarity and consideration for how our subtle energy Reality works to provide real integrated elegant solutions.

Yet this 'incomplete care' is essentially imposed on the public through health insurance plans that virtually define and limit our choices for our own health care. This undermines our personal consciousness to be our own consciously directed authority over our personal health care.

Most 'health plans' will only pay for physiological-based treatments from a physiological view of our health, even though this extremely limited view provides the least likely possibility for clarifying or correcting the real root cause of our problem, which we need to provide an elegant regenerative solution.

Such health care must evolve if we are to ever
have real elegant preventive solutions!

The elegant solution always comes down to attaining sufficient consciousness to live, see and be consciously ahead of our unconscious dysfunctional programming. Only such consciousness allows us to make choices that create real solutions ahead of our unreal, reactive choices that create our problems.

Without clear insight into the subtle energy programming that creates our problems, elegant solutions are not likely to be found. Approaching human health solutions primarily from the physiological point of view is convoluted because it's backward from how humans function and create problems energetically.

Trying to find solutions without knowing the subtle energy choices that are actually causing the problem is like trying to go on a trip somewhere with a *map that does not 'fit the territory'* we are traveling. This situation gives us little knowledge or language to understand where we are, what's going on, and how to get where we want to go, because our *subtle energy 'causes' come into play within one thousandth of a second* from every stimulus in our life, continuously. To be at the *causative level* of elegant solutions requires us to direct our energy to create our solutions *before* we *unconsciously create our problems!*

We have been conditioned to go to the *physiological* doctor when something is wrong with our health. This doctor gives us a *physiological* view of our *physiological* problem, and then suggests some *physiological* treatment using the very limited *physiological* tools of drugs and surgery. Because physiological health care is all about treating physical symptomatic effects, it will be inefficient and ineffective at providing elegant solutions, which can only come from treating the 'cause' of the problem.

When health care services are inefficient and ineffective at providing integrated, conscious solutions – health care costs go up from using more money to try to fix our symptomatic effects that physiological health care alone will never be able to fix! On top of that, public expectations are lowered and Spirits depressed, from seeing too many tragic examples of innocent people who in good faith hoped for elegant solutions from those healthcare providers they trusted, only to suffer the cost of this confusion at the expense of their own personal health.

For example, doctor-related deaths ('iatrogenic' is the word that basically means 'doctor related death') are currently o*ne of the leading causes of death in the United States* (over 100,000 a year). This atrocity creates more fear and confusion about our health care and what to do about our health, which further increases our mental, emotional and physical distress!

Even our current alternative healthcare system often provides only limited, unscientific, loosely integrated holistic conceptualizations of how our body-mind-Spirit Life-force energy functions together. Alternative healthcare options are generally not scientifically supported or convenient to find, which then again tends to further lower public opinion of our healthcare system's ability to provide elegant solutions, leaving us with a feeling that we are not being given insightful, complete and integrated treatment to give us any real preventive and regenerative solutions; physically, emotionally, mentally and Spiritually.

Even so, until recently, most people haven't had many alternative choices in terms of healthcare. But as of this writing, well over a $100 billion a year (which may be much more now) is spent in personal out-of-pocket payments for holistic and alternative healthcare. And, this figure is growing steadily at an increasing rate! This suggests a very high demand for some alternative to traditional health care that provides an integrated view of healthcare services (even though these so-called alternatives using subtle energy treatments are generally not recognized or covered by most health insurance plans)!

Why is the demand for integrative healthcare increasing?

This is probably largely due to the fact that more and more people are realizing that drugs only deal with the symptomatic *effects* of the problem and often actually *compound or create long-term health problems.* Traditional medical approaches are often out of touch with the individual's own intuitive sense of who they are and how they function, especially if they know drugs are toxic and surgery is often a limited, risky, expensive, effect-oriented option that in the long run is usually not an elegant solution.

The best alternative healthcare systems begin with science to track our issues and individualize them into our own unique, integrated personal treatment plan. This enables us to consciously connect the dots from 'where we are' to 'where we want to be' that includes 'how and what we need to do and be' in order to create the real solutions that all Spirits desire.

A personalized profile from infrared scanning reveals our 'drag' on the functionality of specific organ/gland energies or personal powers that make up our Tools. This profile reveals the bigger picture of how certain 'drag' on our Tools of personal powers are misaligning with the Rules (Laws/Ways of energy) to create our life and health problems. This also provides a map of our own personal pathway of recommended integrated behaviors and treatments that support the flow, refinement and regeneration of our Life-force energy from operating consciously aligned with and connected to energetic Reality.

Infrared scans show the 'drag' on specific Life-force energy flow circuits from unconscious *reactive trauma memory* of past unconscious emotionally programmed decisions. With this personal scientific insight we can then learn to *consciously get ahead of this unconscious programming* to feel safe aligning with our truth, then scripting our lines and decisions from that truth. And before we take any new actions to perform that truth (live and in person), we **practice our scenes being able 'to be' who we really are** to replace being *who we are not* (which dishonors our truth in both our words and deeds).

Our organic (organ/gland energy) systems are designed to function in a naturally integrated way to support and regenerate each other providing they are all working without drag so they may spontaneously respond to instantly do what each is designed to do automatically when its energetic function is needed.

Future consciousness-based healthcare systems must include effective solutions and interventions for clearing trauma memory programming issues that create all levels of immense human problems. Such a focus is needed to create any hope for elegant, integrated, mental, emotional and physical solutions to our human problems.

If these unconscious realities that affect our lives in profound ways are not clearly understood and effectively addressed, we cannot possibly ever prevent ourselves from creating and perpetuating our own problems while also limiting our personal powers and our ability to create our best solutions.

Treating symptoms may be necessary for survival in emergencies, but it is merely a short-term, 'band-aid' solution. It would be like an automobile manufacturer who produced bad carburetors. And rather than changing the bad design so they produce good carburetors, they instead created training schools and high-tech research to develop better ways of fixing the bad carburetors that they are creating. They are creating the problem, and then focusing all their resources on trying to fix and survive the problem that they are creating. (Sound familiar?)

If the auto industry solved their problems this way, the cost of cars would be astronomical (like health care) and the cars would not function reliably. We would then need government subsidies to support the dysfunctional designs of the cars. So, the auto industry would need to be subsidized because of its extreme inefficiency. This same type of extreme and costly inefficiency is what occurs when we treat symptoms and ignore the real cause of the problems! [See a humorous demonstration of this point called "The Town of Allopath" at www. mercola.com/townofallopath/index.htm.]

This is why the costs of the traditional health care are so inflated – because it always costs more to fix the problematic effects than to fix the generic causes creating our problems. In other words, we become *less effective* when our unconscious decisions and actions that create our problems remain unconscious!

A short-term view of treating symptoms may *look* productive, because the pain temporarily goes away. But the *temporary pain relief* treatments may be *creating long term problems*. This in itself causes disincentives for even looking for any long-term solutions. Not to mention what happens to the patients looking for temporary pain relief treatments only to become *hooked on the short-term degenerative solutions* (as happens frequently in our current health care system).

Again, we must become conscious enough in our moments of power to understand what is causing our problems and to make choices and take actions that create real solutions. *Consciousness is the only real solution to human problems because it is the only thing that can truly gives us Reality based choices!*

The main reason it has been so hard for traditional healthcare professionals to be more conscious of the underlying causes for ill-health is because their training is almost entirely focused on *physiological factors*. This single-minded approach can only take into account a limited view of the energetic Reality that has very little to do with the subtle-energy programming that determines our physical functioning.

Real and elegant solutions cannot be found by focusing on the 'effect' level of energy, because *we cannot have a solution any better than our clarity for the cause of that problem* (and the cause is always on the unconscious subtle energy level of our energetic existence)!

We simply cannot use the *visible effect – problem-oriented physiological perspective* – to see and understand the *invisible cause – solution-oriented* reality of decoding our subtle-energy programming.

Now, after many generations of conditioning ourselves to accept the physiological view of healthcare as our 'reality,' our dysfunctional healthcare system has succeeded in perpetuating itself to the point where most healthcare professionals don't even think about (or have any options for) focusing on any real, cause-oriented solutions beyond the physical spectrum for their patients to consider in addressing any of their *unconsciously programmed long-term problems.*

Meanwhile, healthcare continues to be run according to the *short-term rules of short-sighted business,* rather than by *long-term rules far-sighted health* that would provide the best personal care. Bottom line driven healthcare runs under the *rules of business* that trend toward short-term dragon 'solutions' which may create huge profits (even though their toxic drug-oriented 'treatments' create long-term health problems). But even that just increases their short-term profits! *This is how iatrogenic problems have made our 'healthcare' system a leading cause of death!*

Cognitive Dissonance

Cognitive dissonance (another energetic Law) reveals yet another huge problematic factor in human consciousness. This energetic Law states that whatever you 'invest in' you will perceive as being 'worth more' – even if the facts prove it to be worth less. (It's kind of like supposing that the longer you wait in line for the ride at the amusement park – the more 'fun' it is.) So, the extent to which we invest our time and energy in *anything* determines our personal value for that thing or person.

When people invest *their entire professional lives* in limited physical perspectives of health or Reality (even if proven to be vastly incomplete) then 'cognitive dissonance' causes them to *overvalue* what is 'unworthy' and to *undervalue* what is more 'worthy.'

Thinking in the mechanical concepts of Newtonian classical physics, we are incapable of conceptualizing the Reality of subtle energy that is the basis of *all* elegant 'cause-oriented' solutions. A very graphic example of how important our subtle energy Reality really is (in the 'real world') is that neither space travel nor electronics is even possible to accomplish using the concepts of classical physics!

So subtle energy quantum concepts of physics are required to even have the *refinement* needed for electronics or space travel! There is a Way that subtle-energy works, and a way it doesn't work, that we must see and understand in order to 'do the math' and be able to follow the pathway to fulfillment.

Newton's theories of classical physics are insufficient for electronics or space travel because they do not even allow for the existence of subtle energy Reality, even in concept (much like our health-care industry does not conceive of problems or solutions beyond the physical realm). Newtonian ideas do not conceptualize energy at a refined enough level to even be able to account for such things as the gravitational effects from planets on a beam of light.

In space travel, for example, this means we are unable to accurately predict where the celestial bodies really are relative to where they 'look like' they are. It takes a more refined view of energy and the math of quantum physics to provide sufficient clarity to get energetic Reality right. The evolving refinement of consciousness for finer and finer levels of energetic Reality is the pathway of change that humans must walk to consciously fully integrate into their total being.

This is surely why William James (one of the fathers of modern psychology who saw psychology as being about consciousness) said that the way change usually occurs is the *old guard dies off*. Change simply happens this way because many people (with the 'dragon' energy in charge) are often not capable of making the evolving change necessary to *transmute* (transmutation being a liver issue) and accommodate to living in a more refined energetic Reality!

> *What we focus on*
> *Is what we get!*

Hypothetical Maps Often Do Not Match the Energetic Territory!

So far, we've talked about 'maps that don't fit the territory.' The medical 'model' is a perfect example as well as our traditional old behavioral psychology that are out of touch with what we now know about the subtle organic energetic nature of individuals. Because, like any science, the old 'models' are based on hypothetical constructs around suppositions the researchers wanted to consider at the time they were made up (which may or may not have been a 'bigger picture' of what really needed to be considered in order to get the answers that could align with energetic Reality).

Hypothetical constructs are made up, of necessity, by scientific researchers. They are constructed as hypothetical imaginary 'as if' suppositions. These are like made-up maps that are *only hypothetical best guesses about the territory.* Since our hypothetical maps might not fit the territory, our hypothetical constructs must be updated at times to keep up with evolved understandings in order to keep coming closer to aligning and fitting with *the true territory* of energetic Reality.

The Dalai Lama was once asked, "What happens if religious beliefs conflict with scientific facts?" He said, "Religion must change." I'm sure he said this because he knows true beliefs must align with and match the energetic Reality we are trying to figure out so conflicting *beliefs* must yield to scientific facts.

In the early stages of any science, when scientists are just beginning to try to figure something out, hypothetical constructs are used to provide 'best guess' scenarios to help make more sense out of scientific data, by either supporting or casting doubt on the hypothesis. If their data ends up fitting their hypothetically constructed 'reality,' it indicates a higher probability of being aligned with Reality.

Hypothetical constructs can be very helpful initially to give the researcher a scenario for what a certain unknown reality might look like. But these constructs can be extremely confusing if or when they are believed and used as a map for operating in the energetic territory where they *do not clearly and completely see energetic Reality*. Then, if and when we act as if our 'hypothetical map' really does fit the territory (when it doesn't), we then create our own *conflicts, chaos and problems!*

Since hypothetical constructs are, by definition, only our 'best guess,' then as 'maps' they may very well not fit the energetic Reality nor guide and direct us clearly through the unmapped territory!

Our insights and solutions can never be any better than the clarity and accuracy of the map being used to navigate our territory! A map that doesn't precisely fit the Real energetic territory is of little value. And no matter how good the map, how clear its details or how well it is packaged – if it is still only a hypothetically constructed reality that does not necessarily even exist – it won't get us where we want to go until it *aligns with, mirrors and matches energetic Reality.*

When we view our world from limited 'hypothetical models' of who we are and how we function, we can have only a limited hypothetical view of Who we are and how we function! In other words, if we don't know who we are, we cannot BE Who We Are!

When researchers do their research, they know their constructs of Reality are hypothetical. If nobody ever imagined these constructs were anything but hypothetical models of what reality might be, there would be no problems created by hypothetical constructs.

However, as time passes after the original research, our hypothetical constructs get printed, believed 'as real' and repeated, to be passed on to many generations. They often become considered and acted upon as if they were actually 'real,' to the point of losing sight of the fact that they are only hypothetical.

A classic example of this is the MMPI (Minnesota Multiphase Personality Inventory), which has been a widely-used psychological instrument (to assist in identifying personality structure and psychopathology). Its model is based on data (with upgrades, I'm sure) from a thousand institutionalized mental patients during the 1940s in Minnesota.

So, in essence, if you take the test, you receive an analysis of yourself that measures how you compare with 1000 institutionalized mental patients in Minnesota in the 1940s (with upgrades based on even more 'hypothetical constructs' about how mental patients' behaviors relate to the test takers). Get the picture?

Then, it goes even further to classify us by comparison with those 1000 mental patients, in terms of certain 'deviant characteristics' that (I guess) are supposed to help us understand ourselves. But we're being compared with *'deviant characteristics'* that are examples of *'who we are not'!*

My experience as a therapist tells me that we *cannot evolve our 'Big Who'* (the Being we are as Spirit Life-force energy) by focusing on and knowing more about the deviant dysfunctional *'little who'* dragon that defines who 'we are *not'! We can't get what we want simply by being clearer about what we don't want.* It may be an effective way to classify *deviants* (defensive reactions) but it is not an effective way to learn to *align* with our Spirit (offensive actions), which is the only real way to 'get points' in life – by learning to be true to our Spirit energies of Love and Light.

No Points for Defense

Anyone who has ever read the PDR (*Physicians' Desk Reference* for prescription drugs) knows that almost every drug in the physician's arsenal of 'treatments' is *toxic to the body.* Drugs create a 'drag' on our Spirit Life-force energy flow to create various types of *short-term solutions,* often at the *cost of long term problems* (this is the classic dragon 'modus operandi'). It would be an illusion to think such toxic treatments could ever provide effective, long-term, elegant, regenerative and sustainable solutions (regenerative and sustainable solutions being the classic Spirit oriented 'modus operandi').

It was reported several years ago that the cost in long-term problems created by these short-term treatment solutions is indicated by figures from the American Medical Association [*www.ama-assn.org/amednews/2011/05/02/prl20502.htm,* from May 2, 2011], which have stated that the cost of treating the side effects of prescription medication is over $76 billion per year and growing (this may be far more now)! This cost per year is just for the drugs that created the problem! This is a negative double-down drag that ensures self-destruction!

As a result, healthcare costs can never keep within normal inflation rates for the rest of our economy because they are out of alignment with regenerative Reality (the Laws of Spirit). In other words, we have a solution that is creating the problem that we are using to try to fix the problem! So, how do you think that is going to work out for creating elegant long term solutions?

When our healthcare 'treatments' contribute to our problems, costs and lost productivity, it ensures the effect is going to be negative. So it cannot rightly be called 'healthcare,' if the overall bottom line Life-force effect is subtraction from health instead of addition to it. Such math would never work productively for any business because it does not add up to regenerative positive effects. Instead it deepens the problem and loses public support by providing outdated, incomplete and ineffective healthcare systems and practices, as opposed to what our Spirits really want.

Traditional symptom/effect-oriented healthcare treatments account for about 90% of our health care costs, even though they can only deal effectively with about 10% of our health problems! This means that 90% of the healthcare dollar is spent on physical treatments that can only effectively treat 10% of the healthcare problems, while only 10% of the healthcare dollar is used to treat 90% of the healthcare problems (unconscious programming) that cannot be effectively treated by physical medicine.

Any system, like any country that over-spends its resources on defense, eventually learns that when they spend excessively on defense, they cannot maintain a positive, productive economy for very long. This is because defensive expenditure is always non-productive and depletes their economic resources (degenerates rather than regenerates). Again, the way the game works is: there are no points for defense.

Until things change dramatically from degeneration to regeneration, we'll automatically create even bigger problems. It's as if the Universe was saying, "If you can't get it at this level of intensity, then maybe it needs to be more intense for you to get it." Could this account for the intensity going on in the world right now and are we finally getting it?

Something worthy of note here: The pressure build-up in the body that happens when we ignore the 'way it works' is not because Spirit is trying to punish us, it's because the Laws of energy are designed to work when they have our attention. But this only works when we are 'paying attention' and are not numb. It is a 'self correcting Universe.' And that's what makes it self-correcting either way. Because when we ignore the pressure, it gets worse and worse until you either annihilate yourself or correct what you are doing. This message is in an old Arab proverb that says: "No matter how far down the wrong road you go – TURN AROUND!"

Spirit 'withdraws' because – if we do not act and listen to these feeling promptings built into our bodies – Spirit energy is diminished because it keeps losing the battle of that decision to the dragon energy! After those Spirit circuits have been diminished, the opportunistic dragon energy can then gain even more strength as it begins to reactively make our decisions unconsciously for us! See the problem?

The primary cause of our human healthcare problem is the *lack of clear consciousness*. This is because only a lack of consciousness allows our most refined human guidance system (consciousness about our Spirit Life-force energies of perception and expression) to be perverted and directed by our dragons. This past unconscious trauma memory projects our thoughts into fears – to be reactively relived in our present, which creates our health problems!

Once we veer off course from our own inner direction, our own intuitive connection with our true Self and our inner sense of knowing, then there is no rational expectation that we will ever be able to find our true Self on that path. That's because our unconscious decisions *keep us disconnected from our true Self!*

However, the good news is that consciousness about energetic Reality as the core of any true healthcare system seems to be gradually getting through in terms of what true healthcare is really all about. This is even true, to some degree, in mainstream traditional circles, which are becoming more accepting of influences from alternative views of integrated health.

This is likely happening because public opinion about the traditional healthcare industry, based on the public's personal experiences with so-called 'healthcare,' is creating pressure on the healthcare industry to become more trustworthy about really taking more 'care' to enhance our health!

This could be achieved by providing integrated healthcare systems with an integrated science that expands our perceptions of energetic health and well-being using concepts that are scientifically integrated into our healthcare practices for improving physical, emotional and mental health.

Chapter 5

Evolving from Past Fears to Present Loves

The Third Dimension: 1/88th of Energetic Reality

Some people believe only in what can be seen, touched and measured. In other words, they live only in the third dimension. The problem with this view is that it limits one to only a small part of Reality – because such consciousness lives only in the third-dimension – which unfortunately is living at the effect (victim) end of the spectrum, often consumed by triggered and reactive emotional trauma memory history.

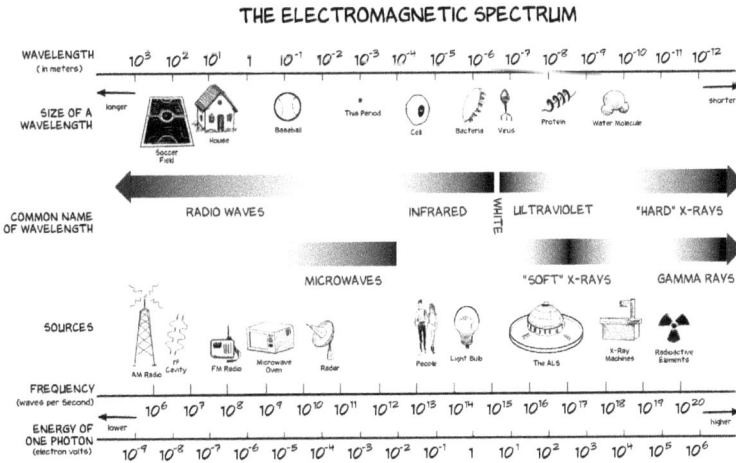

THE ELECTROMAGNETIC SPECTRUM

*The image above gives us a visual perspective of **energetic reality**, or the entire electromagnetic spectrum in terms of wavelengths. This shows the relative size, visually, and the common names, sources, frequencies and electron voltages of various electromagnetic waves.*

The visual spectrum or *third dimension*, according to Joseph Scogna, represents *only about 1/88th of our total electromagnetic spectrum of energy* (despite our many common perceptions to the contrary). Scogna's view is generally accepted by credible scientific sources and many claim *much less* than 1/88th.

We have difficulty perceiving *intangible subtle energy realities* that exist 'beyond the rainbow' of our visible spectrum. Yet, it is the invisible spectrum, comprised of a range of subtle energy beyond the visible, which makes up the other 87/88ths of the entire electromagnetic spectrum of energies that fill in the remainder of the energetic Reality that makes up the Universe!

So, if we perceive, believe and act as if 1/88th of Reality is 100% of all there is – and we perceive, believe and act as if 87/88's of Reality does *not* exist at all – then this distorted view of Reality will continue to create confusion. No wonder the primary human problem is *confusion because our confused distortion of Reality inevitably creates our primary human problem!*

Awareness of our subtle dimensions of consciousness reveal our Spirit Life-force organ/gland energy flow and drag, and gives us clarity into how we create degenerative problems and elegant regenerative solutions. It shows us how to live life so we become capable of eliminating most of our problems.

What happens to us in our life and body is determined by whether we make conscious decisions in our moments of power from following our Spirit's Ways of Love and Light, or unconscious decisions of reactive, confused, projected dragon memories from traumas of fear, force, deception and manipulation.

The question is whether our Spirit has sufficient consciousness and strength to perceive and follow Love and Light in our moments of power, or if our dragon's reactive fears of darkness win over our consciousness to plan, direct and plot our life. This answer is determined by which energy ('dragon' or 'Spirit') is strongest in the moment to make our decisions. It's like the old story about the 2 wolves where the child asks the grandfather, "Which wolf will win?" And the grandfather replies: "The one you feed the most." The same thing applies to the Spirit and the dragon in our game of life. Who wins is all about 'who you feed the most.'

> *So the only real question is: who controls our decisions?*
> *Are we directed by our Spirit's Love and Light, or con-*
> *trolled by our dragon's fears of confusion from darkness?*

If we erroneously think the third dimension is all there is, then this thinking will play into us allowing our unconscious dragons unnecessary power over us. We will remain unaware of why we do what, with whom, where and when – and how our dragons are directing us unconsciously. The force that controls our consciousness, either Spirit or dragon, is the one that will make our decisions that will direct the course of our actions that will guide our life!

The Cave, the Lake, and the Sky of Consciousness

Chinese mythology that dates back over 5,000 years talks about three evolving levels through which our dragons progress under the proper conditions, that they call the *Cave*, the *Lake* and the *Sky*. I have used these symbols to provide a clear, simple model of sequential images that depict the *natural evolutionary pathway of the dragon* evolving through three different levels of our personal evolvement.

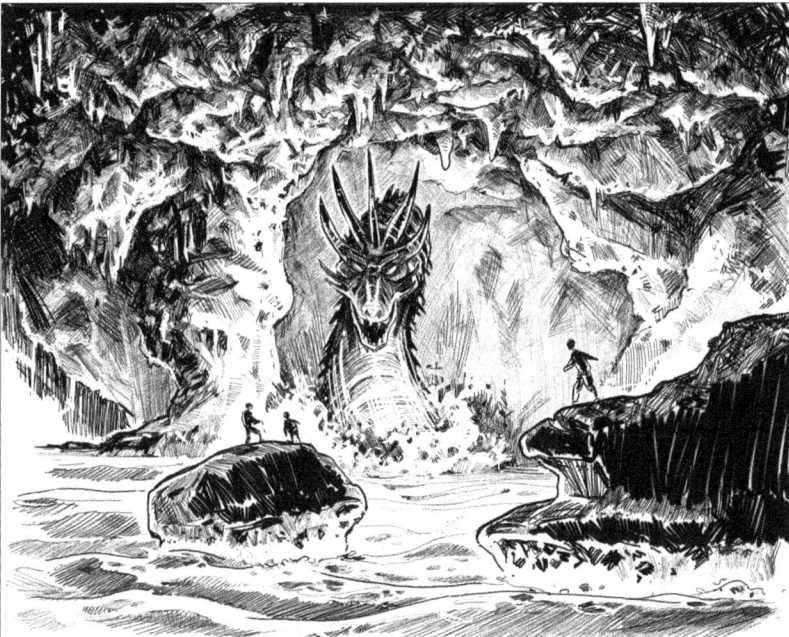

The first ascending path of the dragon evolves from the *Cave* of defensive fears of physical survival where there is no safety, love or trustworthy support. This level is all about defense (where there are no points, as you may recall from our earlier discussions).

The Cave is the dragon's home – a place where fear, darkness and disconnection is 'par for the course' when living in a world of confusion where deception and manipulation is expected and fear is essential just to survive one day at a time. Here, we are always alone, focused on protecting ourselves from everyone in order to survive at any cost, without hope or expectation of trust, love or worthiness!

Within the Cave there are only dragon solutions, derived from past defensive memory of surviving and enduring confusion, deception and manipulation by fear and force one day at a time. So entering the Cave with the dragon is a self-destructive suicide mission! It's like the demolition derby where the last to survive wins, but survival consciousness can only win us physical survival with no hope for fulfillment!

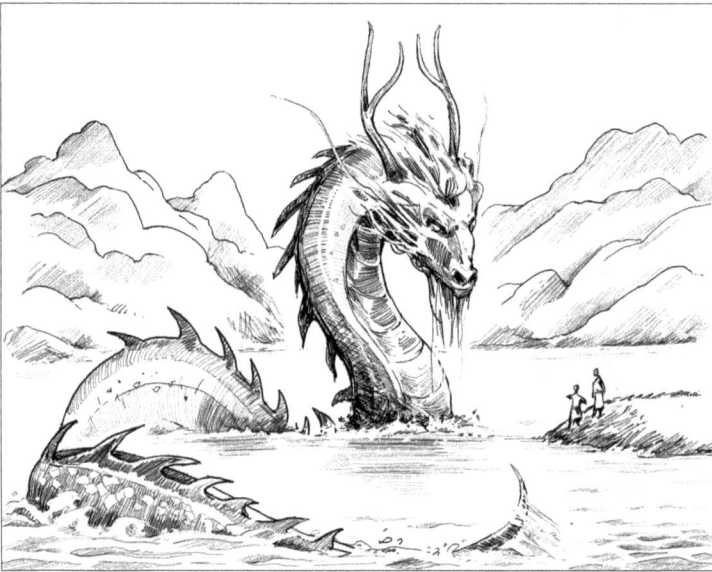

The second level is the 'dragon in the *Lake*.' After gaining the ability to feel safe and worthy of loving our Self and more comfortable owning our Self and our truth, we may enter the *Lake* of our unconscious emotional memory programming to cleanse our Spirit of drag. It is a spiritual 'baptism' of emotional truth. Once we do this, we can get ahead of our unconscious programming so we always have instant access to our own personal programming and powers. When we learn to stay ahead of our dragon's reactions consistently, we can show up authentically, and then learn to live even better with more power.

The Lake represents evolvement toward the consciousness needed for cleansing and clearing our emotional programming so we are more able to stay out of reaction long enough to create new habits of ruling our life consciously without being unconsciously ruled by the reactive defensive ways of drag.

The third level is the dragon in the 'Sky' which can be described as integrated with our Spirit so it serves our Spirit. When we become really good at life, our dragon evolves and more fully integrates with Spirit so they come together in harmony and unity (by using each organ/gland energy appropriately). This is how the power of the dragon becomes directed by the Light of the Spirit, which gives us true power.

Evolution is a process of evolving our Spirit out of the dragon's *Cave* of darkness and through the *Lake* of cleansing so we may ascend into the *Sky* of harmony and fulfill-ment. This is done by aligning our thoughts and actions with the Laws of energy by following the Ways of our Spirit's truth, which releases us from the drag of confusion and fear that creates almost all our problems.

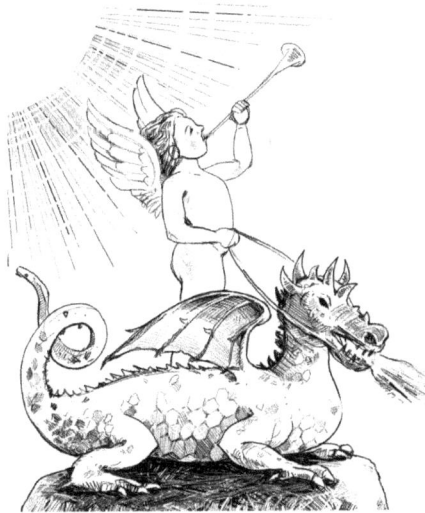

Image re-drawn from an original painting by Radisha.

When dragons are disciplined by the Light with Love effectively, this eventually allows the dragon to feel safe and worthy enough to begin to evolve out of its *Cave* of darkness into the Ways of Light – or the Truth of the Laws. The Light of consciousness disciplines the dragon so our Spirit may gain sufficient strength to consciously get ahead and stay ahead of our over-reactions, over-projections and over-generalizations. We are then able to stay consciously connected to our loving Spirit's Truth which is by its very nature grounded in the light of energetic Reality.

I tell clients a story about *'the consciousness elevator.'* In this story, *the lower the floor is -the darker the game.* The main message of the story is that whenever we go into *reaction* our ascending elevator of consciousness stops and the doors open for us to play life's game on whatever floor we are on (no matter how low it is) to hopefully learn the lessons we need that allow us to get back on the elevator.

Staying out of reactions and consciously connected to our Spirit promptings consistently *raises our 'consciousness elevator'* and enables us to play our game of life in the subtle levels of 'higher energy and evolvement' that always wins more points for our Spirit's fulfillment. Thus, we're able to evolve our Spirit's power into the *Sky* of harmony with the Laws that unites our Spirit's Love and Light to discipline our dragon's dark powers and integrate all our personal powers to focus on fulfilling our divine intent.

When we follow our Spirit's Ways of truth properly and consistently for long enough we raise ourselves to be able to function in the Sky of fulfillment so our imprisoned Spirit is released from 'drag' to heal.

We can only evolve our dragons when we use the proper dose of Love *and* Light at the proper time. Love makes the dragon feel safe to move out of the Cave of darkness, and Light disciplines our dragon with the Ways of Truth that are aligned with the Laws of energy. This is when our Spirit shows up to help us consciously prevent inappropriate dysfunctional over-reactions, over-projections and over-generalizations of Reality that create confusions and problems in our 'here and now.'

In summary, we are designed to evolve from a consciousness of *fear, confusion and reactivity (Cave)* to learning how to connect with our emotional feelings and how to express them effectively and productively *(Lake)*, to using our Life-force energy to perform our life with optimal effectiveness *(Sky)*.

Knowing Whom to Trust

My mother Elsie had a saying, "Time will tell." When we learn to access all of our powers of perception and expression, and perform them spontaneously and continuously with a loving intent and a great sense of humor driven by a quest for the truth, we naturally create and live in a more conscious and refined place of being more readily able to know *whom we can and cannot trust* by clearly observing their Spirit or dragon ways *over time*.

We must know that *attention* effectively reinforces, enables and maintains *whatever we attend to*. Our challenge then is to know what needs to be done to create the regenerative connections our Spirit really wants with those in our life whose presence and deeds are 'worthy' (rather than 'unworthy') of being reinforced by our energy! So, to best evolve our consciousness – we must discern how we live and perform according to how the energetic Laws at play in the various situations in our life. When we do this, we can evolve from living in drag to being aligned with our truth and expressing Who we really are.

As the hippies said, we've got to *"get real"* about what's true in life to consciously *"get it together."* We do this by aligning what we *see and feel* (receiving input), with what we *say and do* (performing output).

When we are more 'real' because we have 'got it together' we will be more believable and trustworthy because we will show up as being aligned with our truth. That makes us more trustworthy, or 'worthy' of being trusted by others to invest time and energy in our relationship. Then we can maintain inspiring and regenerative feelings that fulfill us in our relationships rather than *draining us* of our Life-force energy.

We need this sacred barometer to *keep us aligned with our true feelings* to determine if we can feel safe and worthy just being Who we really are in our relationships by responding clearly and quickly with our truth. We must learn to approach Spirits with the energy of both Love and Light, and to avoid dragon energies (by drawing the line and bowing out) from those that *feel untrustworthy* to have our Spirit's best interests in mind. We need to express what 'works for us' and what 'doesn't work for us (again by drawing the line), and when Spirit prompted, we need to 'bow out' by no longer giving attention/energy to it (so we don't feed it).

As we clear the 'drag' on our Spirit Life-force energy flow, we become more willing and able to follow our Spirit's Light of clarity so we can align with energetic Reality clearer and quicker. Reality's dynamic Laws of energy always create either *regeneration* or *degeneration*, depending on our ability to consciously know and follow (align with) the Laws/Ways in our moments of power.

If you were to ask people what confuses them most about life, you would soon realize that they are mostly confused about simple questions like "Who am I?" and "How do I function?" or "Why am I sick?" or "Why aren't my relationships working?" or "What am I doing wrong to create what's happening in my life and body?"

These are all questions that would never exist in a more conscious world with a clearer, more real and expanded view of Reality that would make the answers to those questions self-evident and undeniable. *These questions are all clearly answered when Reality is viewed in alignment with the Spiritual and natural Laws of energy.* This is because these Laws (when clearly understood) explain the whole 'subtle-energy picture' of Reality and how it influences every aspect of our life.

We are beginning to realize that it is futile to continue to try to stick square pegs into round holes – trying to use Newtonian concepts to understand quantum subtle-energy realities. Reality (when one is fully conscious) is actually much more interesting! No matter how long we've invested in a world that doesn't work, we now see that it is time to give up that old world. We must replace it with an eager willingness to accept Reality and use it to fulfill our divine intent.

When we can accept and perceive a more expanded Reality, we become *students who seek truth* with *pleasure* and are always eager to see the bigger picture painted by the natural Laws of energy!

We then experience firsthand how physics and metaphysics define our energetic creations so we can learn to dance a new and more conscious dance with energetic Reality in Life that regenerates and renews us. Gone are the days when degenerative confusion was our only choice! Instead, with consciousness we can be like the helium-filled balloon that is *finally set free to soar* as we release ourselves from continuous, unconscious, reactive 'drag' on our Spirit Life-force energy flow!

Knowing the specific properties of the dragon and Spirit energies is a huge benefit to *being and knowing who, what and how to choose* to live in the larger, subtle-energy picture (beyond the rainbow of our third-dimensional confinement from viewing only a small fraction of the full spectrum of energetic Reality).

We must always remember that we are Spirits living in a physical body, and our Spirit depends on clarity to stay connected to Reality, so we can align with our powers from the Forces of the energetic Laws.

For example, when a skydiver understands and works with the Laws of gravity, he can use the power of his alignment with the force of gravity to direct their dive to do whatever they want to do during the dive because they know and use this force so it flows *with* them to do what they want it to do. But if the skydiver ever thinks and acts as if gravity does not exist (i.e., believes gravity will have no effect on him – because he thinks he has 'his own reality'), and jumps out of an airplane without a parachute to effectively counter gravity, then this violation of the Laws of gravity will provide immediate feedback, with deadly serious consequences!

This skydiver metaphor applies to **all** the Laws and Ways of Life-force energy because aligning with these laws always define our best performances. Such consciousness spontaneously performed is what we call: "Walking the narrow straight path of evolvement." This is because it is required for all refined performances in the movies of our lives.

Abstract clarity in the moment is essential to direct us, but we still have to 'show up' and perform clearly, quickly and effectively to get points. This empowers us to feel capable of dispelling fear so we know we can handle whatever happens. When we know the Laws that define the mystery clearly, we can then consciously choose to act in alignment with those Laws and Ways and practice their performances and deliver them quickly enough to be believable. The power is in your believ-ability (your ability to be believable) in playing life's game 'ahead of the curve' where all points in all games are won.

We can be ahead of the game in the 'moment of cause' without fear, when we have the clarity to know, see and play life's game in alignment with the Laws of energy and our truth. And of course it helps a great deal when we can also be naturally connected to our Spirit's flow and driven by a loving intent with a quest for the truth and a great sense of humor! That is what personal power is all about! However, it must begin with a clear map that precisely 'fits the territory' so we may accurately plot a trustworthy course that avoids problems and creates solutions.

Our first enemy in life is *fear*, and *until fear is defeated, nothing else matters.* That's because fear will consume all our energy and hold us in our 'Cave' of darkness and confusion. It will also keep us away from the Light of Reality that would allow us to create our solutions where all Spirits can regenerate and be fulfilled by consciously following the Laws of energy. *Clarity dispels fear* and refines 'what we know' and 'what we don't know', which then gives us the power to create our best solutions quicker.

Dragons have all power over all things except the Light! This is why dragons hate the Light. The dragon is the master of darkness and dragons can't play their games of darkness in the Light of Truth. This means dragons are disciplined by the Light of truth and those who are wise to the dragon's ways quickly enough to *stay ahead of their reactive decisions!*

Dealing with dragons is like 'the challenge of the Matador' who uses his cape (representing energetic truth) to keep the bulls eyes focused while performing the right dose at the right time *so we don't get gored by the bull (dragon)!*

When we are in our *Caves* of fear (controlled by dragons) we project our darkness (unconscious trauma memory from within our cells) onto our present by making unconscious, reactive, defensive decisions that shadow and limit our perceptions and expressions that determine the quality of our life.

Only two things get the dragon out of the 'Cave' and into the 'Lake' where cleansing and healing can take place: *Love and Light.* Love makes the dragon feel safe so it can venture forward. And the Light of energetic truth disciplines the dragon so it doesn't overreact, over-generalize and over-project inappropriate trauma dramas!

Twenty-three Dragon Emotions

Our 23 organs and glands' daily emotional functions are essential for optimal performance to survive our physical life and fulfill our Spirit's divine intent. These emotional functions are needed in order to evolve out of the *Cave* of darkness and into the *Lake* of cleansing, clearing and healing by first becoming conscious of how/where our *fears* unconsciously *manifest as reactive drag* on our organ/gland systems.

The twenty-three 'drags' on our emotional perceptions and expressions are defensive in nature and are *reactively triggered unconsciously* (primarily by associations in our present that trigger past memory). Dragons are fear-driven and unless we can get ahead of them – they remain stuck (and we remain stuck *behind* them) with limited ability to get ahead of them appropriately with expressions that clear and heal.

Consciousness gives us access to our personal powers, qualities and functions by aligning with how we are designed to function in order to evolve us from the *'Lake'* of cleansing and healing our emotional trauma memory to clear our view of energetic Reality so we can finally *claim our personal powers* in the *'Sky'* of harmony that fulfills our life effectively by being true to our Self in each and every moment.

Our emotional God-given powers are exquisitely designed for us to 'perceive and express' our personal truth spontaneously, clearly, quickly and appropriately. Any distortions from naturally doing this come from drag on our Spirit Life-force energy flow. This drag is designed to be reactively triggered by unconscious associations and projected instantly into *present* decisions made from *past* trauma memory.

With clarity, we transmute our programmed 'fears' into emotional 'powers' by shining Light on our fears to consciously get ahead of them in the moment. This evolves us through the emotional *'Lake'* of triggered feelings of past unconscious 'trauma memory' conditioning that unconsciously programs us.

Only then are we free to be 'Who' we are as Spirit (Love and Light), and to be finally prepared and consciously capable of doing what is necessary in order to evolve into the *'Sky'* of enlightened empowerment and fulfillment of our divine intent. We'll also then be able to share our gifts with other Spirits, in order to co-create what Spirits desire.

Our 'Lake' of emotional evolvement symbolizes the water-like, 'feeling quality' that our *emotions* represent. And as we evolve our consciousness, we will find ourselves less triggered because we are further ahead of the curve and therefore more able to avoid being triggered.

E-motion is *'energy-motion,'* or the motion of feelings. When this motion is stuck it creates emotional dysfunction. Energy-motions (emotions) are always flowing openly (the way children express naturally), being spontaneously impelled by our perceptions into creative expressions that give us personal power. Or, they are stopped by the 'drag' on our Spirit Life-force energy flow that inhibits us from spontaneously perceiving and expressing our powers.

The big question is whether our Life-force energy is suppressed unconsciously into the defensive and deceptive ways of our dragons – or, if our Spirit's Ways of Life-force energy are consciously *perceived and expressed* so we can make clear, effective decisions and actions in our moments of power. It's all about which energy we are feeding the most. The strongest one **will always be** the one **we feed the most!**

The Universe contains two basic energies we all know about – the *radiating stars and magnetic black holes.* Stars radiate or *push energy out,* and black holes that magnetically *pull energy in and pull mass apart as they reduce* matter into *hydrogen* or light, which is the foundational element of all mass.

These energies either *express forward* (up and out) or are *suppressed backward* (down and in). One is *radiant* and the other is *magnetic*, but both are dynamic in the sense that they are always either spinning energy 'up and out' or 'down and in.' Human black holes (dragons) *unconsciously warp time and space* in such a way that we consciously perceive and express 'there and then' experiences as if they were happening 'here and now.' This is how we all become 'time travelers' without ever knowing it!

Understanding the Laws/Ways of energy allows us to align these two forces onto that straight and narrow pathway that expresses them, so they all dance together. It's like how electromagnetic power is created by performing perfect timing that allows us to do the many things that Spirits enjoy doing.

Not understanding our Life-force powers so we may express the right dose of energy at the right time, leaves us to endure the confusing effects of drag from not knowing and following the energetic Laws of Reality. This is how our 'energetic dance' becomes degenerative, with costly stumbles, shoves and falls.

Without seeing this larger, more refined view of energetic Reality, we see things as black and white, right and wrong, and three dimensional – rather than seeing the bigger, multidimensional picture of how the Universe all works together as one energetic whole. Seeing things this larger way is what our Spirit seeks to learn so we may dance our life's game with optimal power!

Our Defensive Strategy of 'Backward Walking'

Homeostasis is *balanced* Spirit Life-force energy flow, which is needed in order to stay alive (connected to our physical form). It comes in two forms – *offensive* and *defensive*. Both establish homeostasis, but defensive homeostasis is *degenerative* over time, while offensive homeostasis is *regenerative* over time.

The dragon's defensive expressions of 'drag,' amount to what the Native Americans Indians so accurately called *'backward walking.'* This is done when we *don't feel safe or worthy* and it causes our energy to spin 'down and in' to maintain homeostasis and so our Life-force goes 'south' and is consumed by establishing and maintaining survival while in fear, which degenerates our systems. This is how we maintain defensive homeostasis to stay alive (and we do thank the dragon energy for our survival) – but it is costing us precious Life-force energy that will degenerate us over time.

Our Spirit's offensive expression is *'forward walking'* – which is when we feel safe, worthy and free to express our truth and divine intent, clearly, quickly and appropriately so we may be most effective and productive at being Who we are as Spirit Life-force. This is why this kind of homeostasis is *regenerative*.

The dragon is merely the servo-mechanism (an electronic control system) that runs all our reactive behavior from triggered trauma memory of 'drag' on Spirit Life-force energy flow. These dysfunctional habits are by nature reactive 'default' mechanisms designed to operate *unconsciously* from *past* trauma memory – if we are not conscious enough to make our present decisions based on the 'here and now.'

Such reactive behavior can, however, be positive in a life threatening situation, where reactive behavior is very helpful for survival. However, reactive behavior can also be very self-destructive because it time-warps us from our 'here and now' into past memories that cause us to not feel safe and causes others to not feel safe being around us.

The dragon gains control by making others feel unsafe and on-guard, which is disconnecting, dysfunctional and degenerative from too many reactive memories of abuse for too long.

Once we have conscious clarity of our issues and reactive decisions and how they tend to unconsciously repeat our past trauma memory programming, we can then consciously script more appropriate, regenerative decisions in our present that will create the future we desire. Once we are able to do this more consciously, we will be able to replace our 'backward walking' decisions that kept us repeating our past behaviors, with more functionally effective action that give us more personal power.

With sufficient clarity to allow us to align with the Laws of energy clearly, quickly and appropriately, we become spontaneously connected to our twenty-three perceptual inputs and expressive outputs continuously. This gives us the personal power of conscious connection for co-creation with other Spirits to regenerate and process our life effectively and perform in the moment at the speed of light!

This defines enlightened functioning!

Such consciousness allows life to happen with little effort because when we live in the groove of the natural flow of our organ/gland emotional energy (without reactive 'drag' on the clarity of our perceptions and the quickness of our actions in our moments of power) we learn to spontaneously create our most elegant solutions.

Chapter 6

Knowing Your Twenty-Three Spirit Life-Force Energy Systems

Spirits Living in a Physical Body

We must first know and remember that *Life-force energy comes from our Spirit's Life-force* that gives us our mental, emotional and physical powers to run our life! Our bioelectrical Life-force energy flows through our seven chakras, which energize our twenty-three Spirit Life-force energy powers of *perception* (input) and *expression* (output). These powers flow through our 253 binomial (two-way) circuits of organ/gland powers or problems (all with their appropriate symptoms and messages).

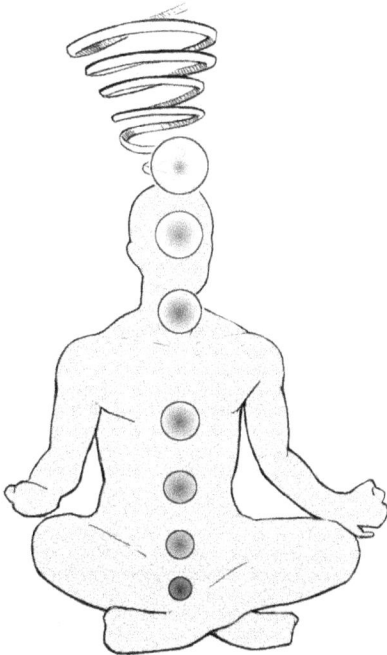

This illustration depicts the seven chakras of our Energy Body that are each designed with different capabilities to interface harmoniously with each other to regenerate and sustain our power.

Our twenty-three organ/gland Life-force energy systems and their 253 circuits of personal power are designed to harmonically integrate with each other to enhance our ability to survive, sustain and fulfill our life by clearly perceiving our options and expressing our solutions. This expression allows us to consciously clear blocked circuits of

drag (trauma memory programming) on our Life-force energy flow –
that creates degeneration, dysfunction, disorder and disease.

Our organ/gland energy systems give us *twenty-three perceptual
inputs* (for how things 'look and feel'). These inputs are then processed
through our *thoughts* (and triggered unconscious *memory* associations)
into our *decisions* in the moment that direct our *twenty-three expressive outputs. These outputs are then designed to* deliver what we say
and do with the energetically *right dose of the right energy in the right
way at the right time* to create our Spirit's desires clearly, quickly and
appropriately.

When this is done properly, these systems spontaneously provide
the *right dose* of power at the *right time* to solve whatever problems or
issues we have – quickly, effectively and productively.

Our system's origin begins at *conception*, when *twenty-three male
chromosomes* came together with *twenty-three female chromosomes* to
conceive our original cell of existence as an individual organ-ism. The
word individual comes from the word 'in-divide' (*not divided* from our
Self). Our organs/glands are all designed to be in 'communion' (not
divided from our 23 emotional perceptions). These powers of perception and expression from Spirit allow us to stay in connection/commu-
nication so we can know instantly what each organ/gland is saying so
we can respond spontaneously and regeneration can occur!

Being 'divided from our Spirit' means we have aligned with our
dragon powers and the many ways of separating and disconnecting us
from life's truths. Separation and disconnection becomes a way of life.
For the dragon, it is way too inconvenient to align with 'what works'
because the dragon is about disconnection. When people's Spirits consciously 'come together' on the usual divisive subjects (politics, religion, etc…), the dragon loses its power. And the dragon does not like
that. This dragon power loss comes from shining the light of clarity on
the *confusions* that it thrives on.

So, when the dragon is 'in charge' it chooses short term degenerative solutions with long term problems. However, doing this continuously bears the cost of degenerating and aging from personal dysfunctions, disorders and diseases on a personal level. And in our world
of nations and communities, it shows up as war, starvation, financial
disasters, etc…all of which maintain dragon energy for long-term
degeneration!

Our body develops from twenty-three pairs of chromosomal (light-body) memory that program our Spirit Life-force energy into twenty-three physical organs and glands, or energy systems, that integrate with our emotional, mental and Spirit Life-force energy functions.

Our body is a holographic mirror image enlargement of our original cell of conception and its twenty-three-based chromosomal format. In other words, it appears that our human functional energetic design is modeled after our own double helix chromosomal (color/light-body) design of twenty-three pairs of memory banks that program our life and body from the nucleus of every single cell in our body.

After conception, our original cell then duplicates itself throughout gestation. One divides into 2 then it divides into 4 that divides into 8 that divides into 16 that divides into 32 that divides into 64, etc. And over a 280-day period of gestation a human being is formed with twenty-three physical organ/gland energy systems that align with twenty-three emotional feeling functions being programmed by twenty-three mental/memory planning functions that direct our Life-force energy to run our life and body.

Our organ/gland Life-force energy is either consciously directed by clear views and thoughts about Reality in the present, or it is unconsciously directed' by triggered time-warps of past trauma memory projected onto our present so we *reactively* live our present *as if* we were emotionally reliving our past.

Our twenty-three Spirit's Life-force energy systems/functions are *integrated powers* designed to fulfill our physical needs and emotional desires. When our organ/gland energies flow freely, clearly and spontaneously, each of our twenty-three organ/gland energy systems spontaneously perceives clearly and responds effectively in each moment to fulfill our needs for safety, nurturance, fulfillment and happiness.

Each system is designed to solve specific life and body problems with certain powers from combined organ/gland energy functions. These powers can either provide emotional perception and expression that creates regenerative solutions, or be overcome with the unconscious reactive drag of trauma memory that causes emotional suppression and disconnection, which creates degenerative problems.

We accomplish regeneration by first having clarity in our perceptions of energetic Reality so we can consciously experience life ahead of our reactive unconscious projections that override clear perceptions and quick appropriate and effective decisions. This point wouldn't be so important except for the fact that unconsciously all dragons intentions are to direct our Life-force energy from their defensive point of view (which in effect creates most of the problems in our life in one way or another).

Uncleared Trauma Memory

Our human systems are designed to work perfectly when we are consciously tuned into our powers. We are designed to operate without drag from anything that would create distractions and confusions. Experiencing continuous drag over time, on the same circuits – creates aging and degenerates our organ energy system causing it to dysfunction from triggered, un-cleared, reactive memories that causes to lose Spirit Life-force, which leads to disorder, disease, and eventually, if the pattern persists, we will *die* because we have lost too much Life-force in one or more organ/gland energy systems.

Our un-cleared trauma memories (dragons) make unconscious decisions in the present 'as if' we were reliving past traumas in our present (by projecting *past memory* to make *present decisions*).

Being conscious of the subtle aspects of our senses and feelings 'in the present moment' and learning to own and use them to direct clear connected conscious thinking and decisions enables us to create what we desire and expect. The perfect plan of Source Energy 'works perfectly' when *we* 'work perfectly' – meaning we need to work the Way we are designed to work energetically in order to regenerate!

Remember, to survive life-threatening situations that we cannot change or escape, God gave us the dragon for our endurance and survival, but these options can only provide us with short-term survival solutions that cause degeneration.

The dragon energy is critically valuable to us in real survival situations, and if we clearly understand its true nature, we can learn to appreciate for what it really is – an *effective essential survival mechanism* (like the oriental world does by celebrating it).

However, if we are continuously traumatized, we activate our dragons' memory of such traumas, and we can become very reactive to unconscious experiential associations that trigger the trauma memory (that reminds us of or 'feels like' similar trauma). When this happens over and over again without resolving emotional stability, we are in effect creating our own personal internal terrorist that will continuously wreak reactive havoc on our life and body until we are able to consciously get ahead of it. Playing the game of life the Way it works is critical! Otherwise, it can be like having a terrorist on steroids living in our body!

When a short-term survival life style becomes too familiar, to the point where we don't know or remember anything else, then the serpent/dragon more easily tricks us into committing 'original sin' (which is going against our Spirit's truth). Doing this continuously feeds the dragon and deceives our view of energetic Reality (just like the story about how the serpent deceived Eve into believing in the dragon's earthly powers of fear and force rather than in our Spirit's etheric powers of Love and Light).

The dragon will sell us anything we will buy! So, when we buy the dragons' inappropriate fears and distorted perceptions (or whatever it is trying to sell us), we go immediately into defense and out of alignment with our Spirit, which divides our Life-force to *counterbalance drag* and maintain defensive homeostasis. This then steals our Spirit energy or power for performing our truth spontaneously and effectively in our moments of decision that determine our personal power.

Our only *real regenerative powers* come from our Spirit's *Love and Light,* which are designed to allow us to find and fulfill our divine intent. Our other *unreal degenerative powers* come from our dragons' defensive ability to endure and survive (and perpetuate) *confusion, deception, manipulation, fear and force.* These negative defensive survival powers are often used to deal with others who are also confused by fear and force, which drives us to do whatever dragons reactively do (once the dragon takes over).

When this happens, the 'not you' (dragon) has taken over Spirit's power, leaving us with our self imposed 'dragon power.' Note: The dragon (being parasitic by nature) cannot create its own power, it can only steal power from confused humans who don't clearly see and understand energetic Reality quickly (and 'buy into' dragon reactivity).

It is said there are three kinds of people: those *who make things happen,* those who *watch things happen,* and those who wonder, *"What happened?"*

Those who have the most power have the ability to 'make things happen' from seeing clearly ahead of the curve and this gives them the ability to create what they want. This ability to make things happen comes from knowing, seeing and being clear and quick enough to take appropriate Spirit actions in the moment.

Those who don't process that clearly and quickly are not able to make things happen for themselves – so they can only 'watch things happen' that are being done by others.

Those who are even more confused process life more slowly (in terms of frames per second) and often don't have a clue about how life works to operate be ahead of the curve, have more difficulty processing life because often when they face issues in life they are only left to wonder: "What happened?"

Having 'drag' on our electrical energy flow is like experiencing static electricity on our circuits of power. It creates confusion. It is a magnetic pulling energy of resistance that goes against our flow (static means 'without flow'). Drag over time causes aging from our processing time being slowed down. Memory of trauma (drag) causes us to not process our physical, emotional and mental toxicity clearly and quickly enough to prevent us from creating a problem that we will then have to defensively endure.

In psychology, conditioned avoidance of negative experiences is called *negative reinforcement.* This is how negative forces gain power over their victims – by instilling fear into them by first traumatizing them, and then offering to not traumatize them anymore if they will yield to being controlled by their fear.

Yielding to control from fear changes our consciousness from one of 'being' to one of 'not being!'

I've always said: "You can't go *north* when you are going *south.*" Aligning with dragon energy changes us from feeling safe and worthy of love to feeling 'unsafe and unworthy of love,' and not feeling like *looking up* to life with plans that are going *north* (connecting with our Spirit's Love and Light).

Enduring is a strong survival mechanism – because as long as we can keep enduring it, we don't have to change it. Dragon consciousness is about *enduring* those feelings of being disconnected, 'unsafe and unworthy of love.' This makes us feel like looking down or going *south* (because we are living life defensively, consumed by fear and confusion).

Amazingly, these two opposing energies literally spin in different directions: Spirit's Light of truth has the feeling of spinning our Life-force energy 'up and out' which creates regeneration because our life is perceived and expressed in Ways that align with the Laws of energy – while the dragon's dark ways of magnetic pull spins our Life-force 'down and in' to create disconnection, degeneration and dysfunction!

Our Spirit's Nervous System

The *secondary* branch of our autonomic nervous system is the *parasympathetic nervous system (PNS),* which is designed to regenerate and rejuvenate all of our organs and glands to heal our physical, mental and emotional being when we feel safe and worthy of love. This feeling also enables our PNS system to perceive and express energetic Reality more clearly quickly and appropriately without triggered *defensive interference* in our spontaneous 'in and out' flow of energy to and from each our twenty-three organ/gland energies!

Our parasympathetic nervous system is primarily activated by sleeping and feeling safe and worthy of Love from trustworthy connections (as well as when we can feel consciously peaceful). Experiencing these feelings frequently allows our entire system to more frequently regenerate itself.

Our *parasympathetic* nervous system is designed to heal and regenerate our entire system, but it can only function most effectively when we're feeling safe and worthy of love or when we are resting/sleeping, which activates our involuntary relaxation response.

So, our body only has access to our Life-force energy healing and regeneration system *when we are not in fear.* Fear is the first priority of our body's energy because of how life threatening it feels to us. There are two branches of our autonomic nervous system, the *parasympathetic nervous system* and the *sympathetic nervous system.* Fear triggers the *sympathetic* nervous system.

So, the parasympathetic nervous system is stimulated by *feeling safe and loved,* and fear stimulates the sympathetic nervous system. This is why it is so important to *stay focused on who and what we love,* without diversions by all the fears that degenerate us. The bottom line is that focusing on what we love inspires, stimulates and will regenerate us and focusing on our fears will degenerate us.

The human system needs to process and deal with its fears clearly, quickly, appropriately and effectively so we can spend as little time as possible focused on our fears, and as much time as possible focused on what and who we love. This directs our creative Life-force energies toward healing and regenerative processes, rather than toward reactive defensive survival processes, which deplete and degenerate our life, body, relationships and consciousness.

The Dragon's Nervous System

Again, the dragon operates its own branch of our autonomic nervous system (ANS), which is called the *sympathetic nervous system (SNS)*. The sympathetic nervous system is designed to *reactivate* 'fight or flight' defensive strategies and actions for instantly surviving life-threatening situations.

Our sympathetic nervous system is famous for 'fight or flight' strategies. It provides immediate physical energy for short-term endurance and in the moment survival decisions for life threatening situations by either fighting the problem or (flight) running away from it!

'Fight or Flight' reactions automatically, instantly and unconsciously take control of all Spirit Life-force organ/gland energy flow (to provide short-term survival) by overriding our Spirit's *long-term fulfillment* functions with reactive *short-term survival* functions directed by past trauma memory programming.

Our 'fight or flight' response is sometimes genuinely needed in the present, if and when we actually need to fight or flee from life threatening situations. And since the sympathetic nervous system is our primary survival nervous system, when it is triggered and controlled unconsciously by the dragon's past memory of traumas in our present experiences – we live our present through our past continuously until we become conscious enough to 'be here now' as much as possible (which is the only way to live in the present).

There may be times when our triggered associated projections of past memory into our present may be appropriate, but there will also be times when it will not be appropriate and that difference has to be figured out instantly and accurately and continuously to stay ahead of the dragons' curves from unconscious triggers.

From the dragons defensive point of view; "You just can't be too careful" and "If in doubt, assume the worst!" This is because dragon energy is designed to cover all negative possibilities. But what we focus on is what we create. So, this negative 'modus operandi' can become a slippery slope if we are constantly consumed by this dragon agenda.

Dragons hate change. There is a big reason why dragons can't and don't even want to consider 'change.' The dragons' primary motive and function is to allow us to survive life-threatening situations we cannot change or escape. And since the only thing they know (and are) is past memory of defensively enduring and surviving certain organ/gland traumas without the power to change or escape them, its primary emotional feelings are driven by a 'fear of the unknown.' Dragons think: "I've survived what I've known so far, so let's keep things the same."

Dragons fear the unknown because it is unfamiliar.

What dragons know is in the past; and what they don't know is in the future. So dragons try to relive their past memory in the present. They project past fears onto present life particularly about change because change is about unknowns and since dragon energy focuses on past memory, the dragon can't change and they only trust what is most familiar! And even if what is familiar is a completely destructive/degenerative pattern, the dragon would prefer that to a constructive/rejuvenative pattern, because it's familiar.

These destructive patterns take their toll on relationships. As I have stated before, dragon patterns have histories of not being able to trust and connect because when they did, they were disappointed in some way. The result is – they fear the future from their distrust of the past, which they project onto the present as resistance (drag) to real connecting in relationships, no matter how safe the present might be.

Dragons fear/hate anything *new* because they are memories of the past or what is *old*. This is also why dragons are not good at coming up with new solutions. But they will never hesitate to criticize anything new, even though they may have no plans or suggestions for doing anything better than what they are criticizing. They may often complain about what is new, by saying things like, "It just isn't the way it used to be," suggesting that everything is worse because it is new – *even if most things are better.*

Dragons seek present times that trigger their past trauma memory, which they may try to sell to us as 'Real' and legitimate in our here and now 'Reality'. The dragon's fears are really 'for us' (sometime from a blind distorted time-warped perspective) to try to 'protect us' from repeating our past (even though focusing on it creates it) in our present and future. Well, the dragon is our past! But if we're not clear enough in the moment, we may buy what they are selling and conveniently remain unconscious about repeating 'what didn't work' productively in our past – and isn't working productively in our present.

So what does a blind, fearful, reactive dragon energy really provide us in terms of what we need most in our life (which is long-term productive and regenerative solutions)? The answer is: "Nothing but survival consciousness." This is because the dragon is not willing or capable of changing its ways. It has no plans to go from doing what does *not* work to doing what *does* work according to the natural Laws of energy because that would mean it would lose its powers to endure and survive without harmony. It does not do this consciously; it just does not know any other way to be. So, it continues to do what does not work unless Spirit's Light can discipline the dragon's dark reactive ways so it may evolve from its 'cave of unconsciousness' to unify with and serve our Spirit's consciousness in 'the Sky.'

The dragon will only come out of its cave if there is sufficient Love to make it feel safe – and enough Light to discipline the dragons' reactive ways as well. Dragon disciplining is what I call our *Spiritual Duty.* This clarity of connection with Spirit consciousness to discipline our dragons with the light of energetic Reality allows us to do in life what makes a big difference in how our life works. It calls for us to show up and perform in order for our inner and outer worlds to work with order and harmony.

Dragons by nature live off the problems that they create! In fact, the dragon plan most often provides nothing but a short-term illusion of any long-term solution of real safety and protection, especially when we consider the dragon's long-term degenerative effects. And like the Mafia's protection racket, the dragon's plan is not really motivated by our long-term protection. This is because the dragon by design (being a survival mechanism) can *only* think *defensively* in terms of its personal survival (no matter what crime or behavior may be involved to do that).

So, when we see this type of behavior we should know that we are observing dragon-motivated and directed behaviors.

The dragon can only see out and it cannot see in. It sees other people's behaviors, but not its own. The dragon sees only 'one-way' because it lacks empathy. It sees only from its own personal defensive survival point of view, which is appropriate for a survival mechanism because survival is not about empathy for others – it's about surviving. But the real question is: "How long do we want to live by just merely surviving?"

Surviving is 'as good as it gets' when we follow the dragon's best ways and solutions, because the dragon doesn't trust – so it can't have the trustworthy connections that would solve its problems. So, it has to stay in defense (which prevents real solutions) and this is why it must endure and survive the problem!

The dragon mechanism is a self-perpetuating cycle of magnetic fear dragging on our Life-force energy, which literally hastens our death by holding us in a continuous state of degeneration by usurping our Spirit Life-force energy source for survival – even if survival is not an actual Reality. This confusion in consciousness causes us to degenerate from dragons supposedly being protective (while actually being and acting like under-evolved Spirits that don't *show up*)!

Our 23 Spirit Life-force Energy System and Their 253 Circuits of Personal Powers

Together, our sympathetic and parasympathetic nervous systems are designed to protect us from things we fear (either real or imagined danger), and to heal us through our love by how we think and act. Because when we are acting and operating from Love with Light, we naturally regenerate all our organ/gland energy systems.

Love and Light go together because they are not whole without the other. Remember that love is the most reinforcing thing there is. So if we try to use only love, we could aid and abet the dragon by being 'too nice' and never disciplining it with the Light of Energetic Reality (what degenerates and what rejuvenates). If we use only Light, there usually isn't enough love and compassion to coax it out of its cave and into its baptism of water/emotions which allows it to drop enough drag' to become *Light enough* to operate in the light (represented as the 'sky' in the ancient mythology).

But when unconsciously triggered trauma memory instantly takes over our organ/gland Life-force energy circuits – "Houston, we have problem!" – a serious energy utilization (survival or regeneration) problem!

Our problems come when our sympathetic nervous system is unconsciously triggered and instantly takes over our entire system inappropriately because the SNS has first priority on our Life-force for survival!

However, since enduring and surviving trauma is the dragon's job (and it loves its job), it loves to keep us in fear and consumed by trauma dramas. In fact, doing this continuously assures and insures the dragon's continuous employment, with a retirement plan that our Spirit pays for. Dragons love doing their job far more than they care about creating real solutions by eliminating what is always causing our problems (simple 'drag on' Spirit Life-force energy flow)! See how there is a 'real' conflict of interest here?

Of course, the answer to the problem is human consciousness evolvement. Living consciously is about learning to be aware of our subtle subconscious organ/gland messages from our various twenty-three organ/gland energy systems and their 253 two-way circuits of powers and problems. Being conscious of each organ/gland energy's *purpose plan, function, issue and trauma* as well as their messages, is what enables us to see and be clear in our moments of power to execute effective actions that prevent our problems and create real regenerative solutions for our life, body, business and relationships.

How our 253 binomial (two-way) circuits of personal power are functioning or dysfunctioning is revealed by our infrared scan that shows which of these 253 circuits are blocked in their flow of power between each other. For example, when the adrenals (the #13 gland with the emotional issue of having the courage to stand up for ourselves) and thyroid (the #10 gland with the emotional issue of taking action to correct personal injustice) work together to express their functions, they provide us with the power of courage to stand up for and create personal justice. When they work in opposition (in drag) to each other (counter-balance) over time they eventually create burn-out from the exhaustion of giving up our personal power of courage (13) and accepting what was not *just and right* for us (10) by not taking action to correct our personal injustices.

The *thyroid* is emotionally designed to enable us to take action to *correct our personal injustices* in the moment they are happening in our life. The *adrenals* are emotionally designed to give us *courage* to meet pressure with equal and opposite pressure (just enough, not too much) so we can face and solve our conflicts with a feeling of pride. The kind of pride I am speaking of is the kind that creates feelings of empowerment (like how you might *stand up for your Self* in the heat of conflict). Standing up for yourself so that you are empowered means aligning your decisions and actions with the Laws of energy.

For instance, when the thyroid and adrenal energies are doing their emotional jobs we experience positive feelings of personal *pride* and *justice* from feeling capable of properly showing up to make things happen in alignment with our Spirit's truth. Together when used properly, these energies have the power to assure our personal justice.

When we don't listen to and act on our Spirit's subtle emotional messages from our thyroid (which will show up as anxiety that tells us to take action to correct our personal injustice), the thyroid function is suppressed. This causes us to continue to endure personal injustice instead of taking action to correct it. Enduring injustices strengthens our blocks/drag on our thyroid-adrenal energy flow circuits, so we learn to just cope with and endure what's not right for us until we are completely depleted and exhausted.

Blocking our thyroid Life-force energy flow; conditions us over time to over-endure, over-adapt and over-accept *what's not right for us.* We do this by taking 'drag' on our thyroid's expression of its Spirit Life-force energy, which is our power to create elegant solutions that are *just and right for us.*

Accepting injustice digs our rut deeper so we feel incapable of expressing our adrenal powers effectively in the moment when our Spirit function is needed to match any pressures instantly and prevent us from being over-powered into accepting what is not right for us (the personal injustices) in our life.

By learning to meet life's pressures with equal and opposite pressure (the adrenal Spirit function) we become much more capable of resolving our conflicts more clearly, quickly and appropriately with the pride of Self-empowerment to achieve what's right, with a loving intent for ourselves and others.

If *not*, we may be blocked (by a triggered thyroid dragon/trauma memory of enduring injustice) from even noticing that we are *enduring injustice* (the thyroid dragon's job). Then, to counterbalance this, we must ignore the pressure (the adrenal dragon's job) created by enduring injustices. We have now created homeostasis by counterbalancing 'drag' to survive what we can't/don't/or won't change or escape.

This is how it works with every organ/gland power. If they are used (as designed) to clearly observe and express their specific feeling energy, they **regenerate** and become stronger. If we disconnect from Spirit Life-force energy for specific organ/gland powers (that are unconsciously triggered by associated trauma memories), the 'drag' on those Life-forces causes those systems to **degenerate** and become weaker.

And as they become weaker, our perceptions of those organ/gland Spirit's Life-forces, their needs, powers and functions become less conscious and apparent. Our organs become 'comfortably numb' from drag on their Life-force so much that we learn to ignore our Spirit's messages easier and quicker.

When this happens, the dragon view is that "It is easier to just become numb (by going unconscious) to our *symptoms and their messages* (even though they will then manifest into our life, body and relationships) and *learn to endure and survive* (one day at a time) with dysfunctions that are causing us to self-destruct."

Consciously we won't even know or experience what the dragon does, as we unconsciously create our symptomatic effects, that either degenerate us from living behind the triggered curves of our unconscious programming, or we learn what they are and how to be consciously ahead of these unconscious curves by knowing and following our Spirit's Ways of truth and personal power!

When Kristy and I teach the Organ/Gland Language workshop, she shares "The Dragon's Song" (a little 'ditty' that she cleverly composed into an irritating combination of two notes), which goes like this: "around and around and around and around," etcetera, sung over and over again on several notes until it is clear that dragons always take us into degenerative circles of repeated patterns that become more and more irritating to Spirits! Maybe dragons can put up with it because of how numb they are, but Spirits just have to do something to change the situation! We stop the song when someone in the group is finally conscious enough to say: "Stop the song!"

This is the lesson of the song demonstration: it's about **turning feelings into actions.** It is to make the point that we cannot ignore 'drag' or irritation, dysfunction and disorder and expect it to just go away – without doing our Spiritual duty – which is when our Spirit *shows up* for our truth. This lesson aptly demonstrated what showing up looks like! It means expressing how we feel as well as acting on those feelings to make our truth known. It means 'walking our talk' so what we *think, feel, say* and *do* all align.

For example, in expressing our adrenal power we must follow our Spirit's adrenal philosophy to learn to meet pressure with equal and opposite pressure. We eventually learn how to resolve conflicts by showing up with our truth and 'owning it' with feelings of pride (worthy 'pride' – the adrenal Spirit feeling). Such performance regenerates our adrenals. If we hold back from *standing up for our truth* (do nothing and say nothing because of drag) we are choosing to *live in this 'drag'* on our truth by pretending not to notice our truth which dis-empowers ourselves from the subtle but definite action of ignoring our Spirit's real truth.

Whether we are ignoring Spirit promptings in our organs and glands consciously or unconsciously indicates our level of drag. If we are unconscious of it, we haven't even begun to do our work. If we are at least aware of what we are doing and yet are still choosing not to translate that into any kind of action to change our situation, then we *are* in less drag than when we were completely unconscious (because we are now to some degree 'aware' of how we feel); but we are still in 'drag' in our ability to express the light of our organ/gland truths clearly, quickly and appropriately regarding that awareness.

In the body, our organ/gland messages must not only be *perceived* but they also must be *acted upon and expressed*. How they are enacted and performed to portray our emotional truths in our moments of power will determine our personal power (just like in the movies). It is all about how we perform and maintain connection with our true feeling Self so we allow our consciousness to function the Way it was designed to function.

Measuring and Tracking Our Spirit Life-force Energy Flow

Infrared science allows us to measure, track and decode Spirit Life-force electrical energy flow patterns between each of our twenty-three organ/gland energy systems. Infrared measures the density of electrons at the junction points on our face (illustrated below) that connect our 253 binomial circuits of human/personal electrical energy flow through our circuits that give us power. This gives us an actual picture of where we are powerful as well as powerless.

Once we are shown our own energetic map that actually fits the 'territory' (which in this case is our unique energy grid), this awareness naturally enhances our ability to feel what we have become so numb to. It allows us a unique way to fill in the blanks about what we have been missing in our lives as well as how to proactively change that situation in each case scenario in our organ/gland language!

These 253 energy circuits underlie all human solutions and problems that come from our various abilities and inabilities to perceive and express our truth spontaneously and effectively. They underlie all human problems because when these circuits are blocked from being conscious and capable of enacting the powers of each of our organ/gland circuits, this creates problems in our life and eventually in our body.

This happens when there is a 'drag' on the circuitry (from triggered trauma memory) that takes us away (time-warps us) from our moments of power!

This causes us to lose our personal power because we are *not there* (our Spirit is not 'in charge'). And when this happens, we are therefore not believable in how we show up and perform our truth in our moments of power. Consistent believability requires us first to be well-connected to our truth and then to perform it consciously ahead of our unconscious triggers that disconnect us from our present. Otherwise we reactively relive our past decision patterns of trauma memory as our present trauma-dramas of our life.

Now we are beginning to see the real human problem – insufficient consciousness for energetic Reality as it always functionally exists in our life. This problem comes from not being conscious of who we are energetically and how our subtle energy imprinting can unconsciously control and direct our entire lives *unless* we become conscious enough to make clearer decisions in our moments of power!

And these decisions are clearly encoded in the language of each organ/ gland energy which reveals to us whether our decisions are rejuvenative and which are degenerative.

We have never been left without answers since the answers have always been within us. We just had to be able to put the pieces together. Each organ/gland is a piece of the puzzle! And there are only 23 of them, so it's really not that hard to figure out once you see each piece clearly and how it all fits together.

Much evidence from many cultural beliefs and practices suggests that we are in the process of becoming significantly more conscious, especially after *December 21, 2012*, when the Mayan Calendar ended and our sun and the planets of our solar system crossed over into the northern hemisphere of the Milky Way Galaxy (after having been in the dark ages of the southern hemisphere for the past 13,000+ years). This marked our entrance into a new age of consciousness that has been variously referred to as the Millennium, the Golden Age, the Age of Aquarius, and the Age of Enlightenment.

A lot has been said about 'junk DNA.' It seems that many scientists have not been able to figure out what 97% of our DNA is, so they have called it 'junk.' Some New Age writers, and myself, believe that at this time, we are now entering a new positive energy field that is beginning to turn on the 97% of our DNA.

This brings us to a discussion about this gland that is often referred to as a 'doorway to another dimension' (which is why it is not included in our 'original set' of organ/glands in this book). Studies have been done since the 60's showing how LSD stimulates the pineal gland. And as a matter of fact, the studies have shown that the pineal gland is stimulated by light!

Having the pineal gland stimulated apparently allows humans to spontaneously become more conscious of energetic Reality. It allows the system to more perceptively be able to process our subtle-energy clearer and quicker so we can have a sharper clarity resulting in a more conscious view of Reality. In fact, the pineal gland literally has an 'eye' with shutters that can open and close like a camera! Life seen in this sharper, clearer way creates and allows us to be more conscious. It's like viewing life with a video shot with more 'frames per second' (FPS) than a camera with fewer 'frames per second' can achieve.

The hippies learned from their own experiences with LSD that it's all about processing what is 'coming at you.' In this situation, it really depends emotionally on how clearly, quickly and deeply you can process your new triggered Reality of *suddenly becoming much more conscious* at many more frames per second. That's because when this happens, previously unnoticed energy becomes instantly revealed. And if we have no concepts to even begin to make sense of that level of experience, this can be awkward at best and confusing to say the least! So how can we even begin to make sense of our experience?

It's a good thing this language has always been inside of us! Short term, it's like learning any other language because there is some effort involved to learn who you are and how you function. But long term – once you know the language – your life can never operate at the old level of consciousness again. Once you've 'seen it', you can't 'un-see it.' It's subtle, but immensely powerful.

So if (like a sunrise) our entire planet is literally moving into a brighter and more enlightened era, then our conscious awareness of our energetic Reality is now expanding rapidly into what some have called "The Quickening." Because of this new and expanded awareness, everything is suddenly becoming much sharper and clearer to us. Can you see how this will move us toward a future of more refined dimensions of consciousness? With this new light dawning on us, we are all being compelled to expand our consciousness in order to adapt to our new dynamic world.

But remember, it's how we *process* our consciousness for our new Reality that makes all the difference between a 'bad trip' and a 'great trip' in life that provides an enlightening and fulfilling experience. This difference comes down to our ability to feel safe. It's also about being open enough to receive and perceive our subtle energy clearly, so we can better conceptualize a whole new expanded view of energetic Reality.

The personal subtle energy concepts used in this book have already proven extremely helpful to thousands of my clients by helping them to recognize the bigger picture of their challenge. These ideas have helped them conceptualize their solutions so they can see, understand and do what it takes to stay ahead of the curve of unconscious reactively triggered past trauma memory in life during their moments of power!

Our life's 'movie' performance (which boils down to our performance in life) is about *how* we express ourselves (body language and tone of voice), which accounts for about *90%* of our effectiveness. Whereas *what* we express (the content, script and words we choose) only accounts for about *10%* of our effectiveness at almost anything we do!

So *'how'* we show up is almost everything and *'what'* we say doesn't really matter much, unless we also have great *'how' (bad 'how' is a bad problem)!* So of course it takes *both* 'how' and 'what' for us to perform so we get what our Spirit really wants!

Just as we speak and express with our voice, our organs and glands speak also in coded messages that relate to their unique feeling/ energy function they are designed to accomplish as their purpose. For example, the purpose of the thymus is 'protection'; the purpose of the heart is 'harmony'; the purpose of the colon is 'elimination'; etc. for twenty more organ/gland energy systems to be outlined ahead.

All of our organ/gland systems are designed to help us perceive and express certain aspects of our life where certain Spirit Life-force energy is needed to connect us to that part (organ/gland energy) of Who we are as Spirit beings in a physical body. These circuits are each designed to help us direct a path for Spirit Life-force energy to regenerate us and create a more fulfilling daily life.

What gives us maximum power is being consciously connected to our Spirit's truth spontaneously, at the speed of light. And if we are able to perform that truth in all the moments of our lives with a Mona Lisa smile, a loving intent, and a quest for the truth, while keeping a sense of humor – we won't be taking things in our lives too personally or too seriously – and that's when life gets really fun!

Where we focus our attention will create what our lives look like. Performing the movie of our life with a *great sense of humor and a sense of detachment* (from what is least important) is critical in relation to where we focus our attention. Many absurdities happen in life (that can end up providing our greatest and most profound lessons), which may at first be hard to take but if we can learn to have a sense of humor about them they become a lot less difficult.

Humor can also allow us to be more easily and readily heard by making it the "spoonful of sugar that makes the medicine go down." It can also allow our Spirit to shine by making any situation (no matter how difficult) a lot easier to deal with by just adding humor to our Spirit's Love and Light!

Most of our problems are essentially created by trauma memory making unconscious decisions for us that create 'drag' on the flow of our Spirit Life force energy functions of perception and expression to create solutions. These solutions have the potential to expand our conscious connection with our truth, which sets us free to be true to our Spirit, so we are better able to 'show up' and perform our truth spontaneously with more refined perceptions and expressions.

Our twenty-three organ/gland energy systems have always used their natural language to encode our traumas and lessons into our organ/gland memory banks as part of a specific plan for how particular organs' operate and function by perceiving and expressing their specific purpose. Our consciousness for our organ/gland systems must be able to allow us to avoid, or at least get ahead of, making unconscious disconnected triggered decisions that are projected from our past trauma memory.

Our Performance Tools: Our Twenty-three Organ/Gland Energy Systems

Our mechanism for accomplishing our magical life task of *maintaining rejuvenation* is contained within our twenty-three organ/gland energy systems and their 253 binomial circuits of *powers* that reveal how we function in each organ/gland's physical, emotional, mental, and Spirit Life-force energy performances.

Problems are created when our circuits are blocked by the triggered 'drag' of trauma memory on our Spirit Life-force energy flow. This drag prevents our Life-force energy from providing the personal power that is possible when Life-force spontaneously flows through our 253 circuits to solve specific energetic problems in our life, body, business and relationships clearly, quickly and appropriately.

Our 253 binomial circuits represent what we may call our 'powers and problems language' that conceptualizes how our Life-force energy functions and dysfunctions for health or illness. These 253 Life-force energy circuits reveal our degenerative coding of disease, disorder, dysfunction and degeneration – physical, emotional, and mental issues mirrored on different levels of energy density.

All electricians know about the term 'electrical resistance.' This is what builds up into pressure on the circuits enough to cause them to 'burn out' from the heat of resistance. The same is true about the Life-force energy circuits in our bodies. These circuits either flow spontaneously or they are blocked by drag from triggered trauma memory (that builds up negative magnetic pressure that blocks the circuits over time). When too much resistance (to our flow with energetic Reality) occurs for too long, the 'drag' devolves our Life-force energy and takes over our personal power to become our version of the 'not you.'

These blocked or partially blocked Spirit Life-force energy flow circuit patterns reveal our most basic sub-conscious energetic programming for how we approach life (in the ways we perceive and express each energy), and the drag on flow that manifests as problems from how we *resist* really living our truth!

Our Twenty-three Spirit Life-force Organ/Gland Energy Functions

The following section details each of our twenty-three Spirit Life-force organ/gland energy systems and their functions. It deals with how each organ/gland Spirit Life-force energy system mentally, emotionally and physically either processes its past trauma memory into regenerative health; or projects it into our present decisions/performances to create *d*egeneration, *d*ysfunction, *d*isorder, *d*isease, *d*eath and *d*ying. (Notice all these words begin with a 'D' because they all represent the effects of '*d*rag' on *Spirit Life-force energy* flow from continuously triggered un-cleared *reactive trauma memory*.)

Think of each of these twenty-three organ/gland energies as resonating at a different Life-force energy frequency, each with its own specific *purpose, plan, function, issue* and *trauma*.

These organ/gland energies, when integrated consciously and effectively to complement each other are designed to be regenerative and productive by expressing and perceiving our 253 circuits of refined personal powers of conscious mental, emotional and physical discernments in our moments of power.

When we become conscious of how, when and where our unconscious programming is creating a 'drag' on our power – it instantly loses its power! These are the 'ah ha' moments of enlightenment that enable us to consciously get ahead of our unconscious habits before we enact them. This allows our organ/gland powers to be free of being unconsciously and reactively directed, to be able to be consciously directed to do what each organ/gland energy is designed to do to fulfill our mental, emotional and physical needs and desires, which ultimately is what rejuvenates and regenerates our health on all levels of our life.

Each of our twenty-three Spirit Life-force energies are briefly outlined below in terms of their positive Life-force energy functions, their negative unconscious dragon survival functions, and their specific un-cleared trauma memory issues. Then in Chapter 2 (in "Know Thy-Self" – Volume II), we will go through each of the organ/gland energy systems again as we look more deeply at them in terms of their effects, or symptoms, that result from drag on each of their functions. We will also provide more details on how those symptoms are programmed in each of us.

Some of the words describing these innate organ/gland energy functions are the same words Joseph Scogna used in his book, The Secret of SAF, to describe these natural energies/feelings. I use these words (for the same reason Joe likely used them) because they provide the most appropriate organic descriptions of these organ/gland energies. (See my Amazon Consciousness Bookstore at: *http://DGAllenPhD.com*.)

1. Thymus Spirit Function - Our Protector

Our Thymus Spirit Life-force energy is functionally designed to provide us with the appropriate amount of aggression needed to protect our Self. It is essential to feel safe and capable of expressing the proper amount of aggression needed without *feeling unsafe to use aggression effectively.* When properly used, aggression allows us to feel safe *in knowing* that we can express the appropriate amount of aggression needed to protect our Self. This energy when working properly is like immunizing ourselves against outside invading forces, such as emotionally toxic relationships, by being able to clearly and quickly act to avoid or neutralize whatever feels like it is going *against* our Life-force.

The thymus dragon nature is about *re-acting* triggered associated trauma memory in our present energetic Reality as reactive decisions and actions to protect us from aggressive actions against us. These are very functional in life threatening situations and very dysfunctional in life especially in relationships.

When we are consciously aligned with our thymus Spirit Life-force energy, it naturally performs the right dose of aggression in the right way at the right time in our moments of power to allow us to feel safe within our Self. Safety is the primary factor that keeps us out of defense and is essential for all other organ/gland functions to operate effectively.

Feeling safe is absolutely imperative for our systems to work regeneratively. *This is why the thymus is so critically required and why it is number one in the 'degenerative order' of importance for survival.*

Above all, we must be able to stay out of inappropriate reactions where the dragon's defensive behaviors take over, because these reactions trigger other people's dragons. This then causes almost all our energy to be directed and consumed defensively – so it can't be used to regenerate us. And of course this causes us to degenerate our system energies.

The thymus dragon enters the picture when thymus Life-force energy is forced to endure feeling unsafe and overpowered by more aggressive forces (often parents). This can happen, for example, when a child experiences being aggressively overpowered and/or being punished for taking aggressive actions to protect him or herself. At this point, we take on a programmed, conditioned 'drag' on our Spirit's thymus energy of aggression that is designed to defensively protect us by either holding back our aggressive action or overreacting with them, in order to try to avoid over-aggression from more aggressive forces.

When we need to aggressively protect ourselves, our dragon may either *reactively endure and survive not feeling safe* to protect our Self; or become *overly reactive and aggressive* by over-protecting our Self now from what we couldn't protect our Self from then, as if we were reliving a past memory.

Also, it is important to note that overreacting aggressively can have ongoing consequences. For example, if we are familiar with being around threatening people, then we are more likely to assume new people will also be 'threatening.' So we will act 'as if' they're threatening, which will most likely make them feel defensive and therefore they'll feel more threatening to us (justifying our need to be threatened by them). So, when we act as if they are threatening to us, they are much more likely to act as if we are threatening to them. In other words, aggressive overreaction, or defensiveness creates more aggressiveness and defensiveness!

When these unconscious triggers happen, it's very difficult, if not impossible, to notice (in those reactive moments) that we are *reacting inappropriately* in terms of what is real in our *present* energetic Reality (relative to our *reactive aggressive actions*) and they certainly won't create the future our Spirit desires.

These reactive trauma memories can create long-term problems of feeling unsafe and being unable to maintain appropriate, aggressive action relative to what we may feel is needed to protect ourselves. These reactions can result in an *over-activated immune system*, when the body is constantly being triggered to reactively protect us *in the present* as if we were reliving our fears from a *past* memory that is now being experienced as a *time-warped projection we are living in our present* as if it was real *now*.

The emotional function of the thymus is designed to protect us from outside invading forces by first feeling safe to be sufficiently aggressive to be able to protect our Self. In other words, we are designed to protect our Self with aggression, from those who are against us, and to also feel able to create our own safety through our own powers. (This is the main emotional function of our thymus energy.)

The thymus dragon memory of enduring and surviving feeling unsafe diminishes our emotional perceptions and discriminations for appropriately feeling safe or unsafe in our present life because of our projected memory creates a fear of repeating past unsafe situations we could not change or escape.

Remember that all organ/gland issues have a 'too much' and 'not enough' component to consider when making decisions because the 'too much' and 'not enough' for each organ/gland is dragon territory. In the case of the thymus, the 'drag' we take on to survive not being or feeling safe, causes us to numb our sensitivity so we don't accurately experience safety or the lack of safety. This is how aggression/ safety issues become either 'too much' or 'not enough' safety and/or aggression.

So in other words, *inappropriate dragon aggression* usually looks like too much or not enough aggression, while appropriate Spirit aggression is always the right dose of aggression, in the right way, at the right time.

The conscious, elegant solution for thymus energy is to clearly and quickly discern between what or who is safe and unsafe; and to not act safe when we do not feel safe … or *act unsafe* when we **are** *safe.*

Un-cleared trauma memory of enduring feelings of being unsafe creates thymus issues from not feeling able to express our thymus Spirit Life-force energy (appropriate aggression) to create our own feeling of safety by using proactive measures to feel safe.

Not being able to be true to our Self and feel safe to be Who we really are (so our nervous system can relax and function effectively) forces us to *defensively* endure and survive feeling unsafe. This is an unsustainable, degenerative strategy that will inevitably create thymus (immune system) health problems.

2. Heart Spirit Function - Our Lover

Our heart's Spirit Life-force energy function gives us harmony and synchronization through the powers of Love – our *only purely positive Spirit emotion* [capitalization refers to Spirit Love]. The operative word for Love is 'accept' because if we don't feel 'accepted' we don't feel loved. The Way Love works is that our Spirit naturally Loves, and our dragon naturally fears and is skeptical of those who make us feel safe and worthy of Love.

Loving, accepting behavior is Who we are as true Spirit Self – so our Spirit is *always* clear and *loving in how we connect with the real essence* of Truth as defined by the Laws and Ways of energy – *if/when* our Spirit has control over our decisions. If our *Spirit* does not have *conscious control* over our decisions and actions, then our *dragons* have *unconscious control* over them when the dragon operates as our *default.*

Loving acceptance creates a feeling of being loved or accepted for being Who we really are as our true Self. This synchronizes with and attracts Spirit-driven people who can do what is necessary to be and create Love, to be worthy of real harmony, which requires Love. Thus, being accepting and feeling accepted (Love) together creates synchronized harmony. This is the main emotional function of our heart.

The heart dragon memory of untrustworthy love dims and confuses our emotional perceptions and discriminations for who has what it takes in terms of trustworthiness in Love, versus choosing those who are not trustworthy with the heart in Love. The primary issue with Love is to feel accepted and to lovingly accept what we cannot change from a sufficient distance that we can still Love the process. So feeling *un-accepted* is the same as feeling *un-Loved.*

The reason *Love and Light always need to go together* is because *one without the other does not work. Real Love is always aligned with the Light of energetic truth.* And if it is not, then a form of 'dragon love' is identified as it takes over by reinforcing, enabling and maintaining *self-destructive* behaviors that degenerate us in the long term.

Indications of when this dragon energy has taken over are when we feel too afraid to speak our truth. Or, it can manifest when our 'truth' is skewed somehow (not energetically correct) and we speak that instead. Either way, we are not aligned with energetic Reality because we either do not know it (because we are not connected to it), or we are willing to speak about generally anything *other* than the energetic truth because of *how inconvenient it is.*

Knowing how to avoid *reinforcing, enabling and maintaining degenerative behavior is consciousness. Knowing it and enacting the* straight and narrow path that integrates Love and Light in what is called 'tough love.' It is about shining the light of energetic truth (when Spirit prompted) on situations that can benefit from it long term. Walking this path of the Laws of Light through the Ways of Love is 'tough' (but the only thing that really works).

The 'drag' on our heart energy is about us 'taking on drag' to counterbalance disharmony and deny our need to feel loved and accepted for Who we really are. The heart dragon allows us to survive the disharmony of not feeling loved and accepted by acting as if everything is fine when we don't feel loved (which is what we call 'denial'). This numbs our sensitivity for accurately experiencing and knowing the feelings and actions of being loved and not being loved.

Remember, 'too much' and 'not enough' are *both dragon problems* operating from dragon territory, which come from triggered unconscious *reactive emotional memory* and habits. When we feel safe and worthy of Love in our heart with a clear concept in our mind about what Love is and is not – we will no longer 'try to feel' we are being loved (when we don't really feel we are being loved). And we will no longer 'feel unloved' by those who really do love us when they have loved us all along.

Dysfunction in our relationships results from continuously triggered memory of not feeling we are loved and accepted, without being able to communicate our truth to clear and heal our circuits by feeling loving acceptance when we really do 'show up' for Who we really are. We only heal by getting real in the moment with our true feelings and learning to live there and then notice who loves us when we are being our genuine selves.

The conscious, elegant solution for heart energy is to learn to quickly perceive who really accepts us by clearly discerning who makes us feel accepted (Loved) and who does not. Doing this well allows us to be able to discriminate clearly between harmony, with love and acceptance versus disharmony from denial of love without acceptance.

How we feel about Love, is how we act about Love. If we don't feel loved, we feel unaccepted and then we create a *body language image* of someone who doesn't feel loved. When this happens, we can't figure out why nobody loves us (except for those who *don't feel loved* – who identify with us). And these are the same people who *don't know how to love* because they've *never **been** loved!* See the problem?

Our first solution must always be to develop our own *loving acceptance of our Self.* We do this by realizing that how we feel about our Self sets the course for everything else and the better we feel about our Self the more we can help others feel better about their Self.

To do this, our behavior must reflect an attitude of being worthy of Love (and NOT act as if it is okay to be treated like we are *unworthy of love*). This way, we *always feel accepted by our Self* and those who accept us for being Who we really are as Spirit. This Self acceptance empowers us by knowing that we cannot give out of an empty cup. But if ours is inherently full through Self Knowledge, we are free to accept others with the same grace that we accept our Self.

Spirits act like Spirits and dragons act like dragons. And since we are influenced by both of these energies within ourselves, our long term Spirit solution is to *get closer to* and *more connected with* those who harmoniously love and accept who we really are *(which regenerates us)*. And it also means to *get further away from* and less connected with those whose behaviors create continuous disharmony in us that clearly shows they don't really love or accept us *(which degenerates us)*.

As stated before, inappropriate 'dragon love' is about too much or not enough 'love' for what is and is not trustworthy of Love. 'Spirit Love' over time discerns between real loves that synchronize with acceptance for what is worthy of loving harmony, from those who create disharmony who are not real and are not worthy to sustain real Love.

Healing our hearts comes down to perceiving who really loves us and then expressing the right dose of love, to the right person, in the right way, at the right time. The stuck energy of un-cleared heart trauma memory creates heart issues from enduring disharmony, usually from *not making discerning choices* between those who *really love and accept us* for who we are and *those who do not*.

3. Colon Spirit Function - Our Eliminator

Our colon Spirit Life-force energy is designed to give us the ability to *eliminate what we hate that no longer nourishes us,* and the consciousness to know the difference between what we must eliminate that no longer nurtures us – and what has worthy nurturance value that will help us achieve success in our life.

We also must *eliminate* habits of *holding on* to things we really don't want or need that only hold us back from achieving what our Spirit really wants. When we eliminate what doesn't nourish us, we detoxify and get rid of toxic feelings of 'drag' (which prevent us from eliminating what does not nurture us and becomes a vicious 'down and in' negative spiral of drag).

The *elimination of what does not nourish us* is a major achievement in our life (and body) by freeing us from the drag of holding onto what we don't need or want any longer. When we eliminate the 'crap' that holds us back, we feel lighter and more compelled to move forward toward what nurtures us.

The colon dragon comes from our colon Life-force energy being defensively programmed with 'drag' from the *memory of having to 'endure what we hate' that does not nurture us.* The colon dragon creates an energetic drag on our ability to consciously perceive and *discriminate between what nurtures us and what is toxic* to us that we hate and need to eliminate.

If our colon Spirit Life-force energy holds the drag of past trauma memory from not being able to eliminate what we hate, this memory creates an unconscious 'drag' on the nature of our colon Spirit Life-force energy to eliminate what we hate – to achieve optimal power.

If we don't know what we hate and/or, we are *unable to eliminate what we hate* (what does not nurture us), then by default we hang on to and *endure hating what does not nurture us* – as if we had no power to make any other choice. (And when this happens: "Hello, colon problems!")

Such behaviors are often associated with *colon dysfunction* and *anal-retentive personalities.* These characteristics tend to *endure and hold on* to things and people who are toxic *to them* and *do not nurture them.*

The emotional function of the colon is designed to eliminate the mistakes of 'love' (that we grow to 'hate') by eliminating what is no longer nurturing us. In other words, we are designed to feel hate **as our signal** to expel what is toxic or non-nurturing by discerning what is nurturing, versus what is toxic and needs to be eliminated. (Otherwise we enable and maintain toxicity.)

Eliminating what does not nurture us inspires and regenerates our colon Spirit Life-force energy detoxification function. Our colon dragon memory of having to endure and survive what we hated dims our conscious perception and discernment for noticing quickly what we hate and what no longer nurtures us. The defensive function of this dragon is to allow us to endure and survive toxic situations that we really cannot change or escape and must do but only for a very short time or we feed the dragon.

We take on colon 'drag' to endure/survive physical/emotional 'crap' rather than eliminating it when it is possible. Enduring non-nurturing crap causes us to numb our awareness of crap (and our motivation to eliminate it). The conscious, elegant solution for colon energy is to clearly and quickly discriminate between crap and nurturance, and then eliminate what does not nurture us before it drags us down.

The un-cleared colon memory that creates colon problems is memory of having to 'endure crap' which we defensively deal with by learning to 'not see crap' (even if we are wading in it).

We do this by taking on drag (from colon dragon memory of enduring crap we hate) on our colon Spirit Life-force energy thinking and feeling functions in order to disable our ability to express our colon Life-force energy. Otherwise, our colon Spirit Life-force energy function would spontaneously eliminate the non-nourishing crap from our life (by *choosing* what needs to be eliminated, and then *eliminating* it).

Being unable to perceive or express our colon's Spirit Life-force energy so we can notice and eliminate what does not nurture us – forces us to defensively endure toxicity as a strategy – which is an unsustainable and degenerative colon dragon strategy that will inevitably lead to colon problems.

4. Stomach Spirit Function - Our Nurturer

Our stomach Spirit Life-force energy is designed to give us the ability to nurture ourselves. It is the consciousness to know that nurturance is essential and be able to feel happy about nurturing our Self as if we deserved to be nurtured. The reason is that if we don't nurture our Self, we have less to offer others!

The stomach and small intestine nurturance/nurturing function is designed to nurture us by digesting, dissolving and assimilating our food and life circumstances into the fuel/nurturance and happiness needed to effectively run our vehicle (body) and perform our life using all our Life-force energy systems and functions. Nurturing our Self often requires reversing old habits of 'enduring and surviving not being nurtured' and/or not nurturing ourselves or others.

Our feelings of being nurtured give us the ability to feel safe to open up more to see and feel more quickly to better discriminate between what looks and feels nurturing to us and for how long is it nurturing – and what is not nurturing – and then choose what nurtures us and avoid what does not, much like we would choose what to eat at a smorgasbord. We nurture ourselves by taking in only what really nurtures us.

The stomach Life-force energy functions uses physical chemistry and emotional enzymes to break down food (problems) into nurturance by digestion to dissolve food (problems) into small enough bits to be a solution that it can be assimilated through the cell walls to be absorbed into our system as nurturance.

The stomach's Life-force energy is designed to confront and break down our food (circumstances and problems) into nurturing solutions in our life that create happiness. It does this by using emotional and physical enzymes to confront and digest these circumstances and food into small enough bits to dissolve our problems into nurturing solutions that can be assimilated and absorbed into our body and life to nurture and sustain our Life-force energy.

On an emotional level, our stomach Life-force energy is designed to allow us to see, feel and choose or 'take in' what is nurturing to us, by following our stomach feelings from 'nauseous' to 'nurtured.' And, over time, paying close attention to this 'stomach discernment' is the pathway leading to what makes us happy – because we are more often than not choosing to be nurtured rather than nauseous!

When our stomach circuits are consciously open to their natural feeling perceptions and expressions of happiness and unhappiness, we are better able to spontaneously know what problems we can digest, dissolve and (which ones we cannot) assimilate into refined enough solutions to nurture our life and body to feel happy.

The stomach dragon enters the picture as memory of trauma to our stomach Life-force energy of enduring without physical and/or emotional nurturance. This causes us to take on 'drag' on our stomach circuits in order to numb our feelings of hunger and unhappiness from not feeling or being nurtured.

To survive without nurturance, we take on drag on our senses and feelings for refined taste to discern nurturance and happiness in our life's choices. And then, because we are without nurturance we defensively learn how to better endure and survive by 'drag' on nurturance discernment (e.g., eating junk food) for short-term happiness (nonnourishing food and relationships). (And when we do that: "Hello, stomach problems!")

If stomach Spirit Life-force energy holds un-cleared/unconscious trauma memory of past indigestible (non-nurturing) experiences that we could not solve and assimilate into happiness – then these uncleared memories of *indigestible situations* (when triggered) cause a 'drag' on our stomach energy flow. This is a 'drag' on the energy that powers our ability to digest, dissolve and assimilate our food and life into nurturing solutions. See the problem?

Triggering this stomach memory of enduring and surviving without nurturance and not being able to digest, dissolve and assimilate difficult life experiences, causes us to project past time-warped decisions and actions onto our present as if we were reliving our past memory of having no choice (in our present).

If the stomach dragon can sell us this projection (as being true in our present) this means that we must try to get nurturance *from those who are not capable of nurturing us.* (Warning this may give you ulcers!)

Trying to do what can't be done only creates the need for more 'drag' on clearly seeing Reality and expressing our 'emotional enzymes' to confront hopeless situations that our stomach Spirit is not happy about. So we must either 'digest the indigestible', or 'throw it up' and get rid of it.

Because, if we can't dissolve our problems by breaking them down into nurturing solutions that resolve things, then we will not be able to really 'stomach' the problem – because it is toxic to us or provides us with no nurturance.

The emotional function of the stomach is designed to provide us with *discernment* for what is most and least nurturing to us that makes us happy or unhappy. In other words, we are designed with the ability to make clear, quick discriminations about *what nurtures us* and *what does not,* and then learn to choose and follow what is nurturing (because it can be digested, dissolved and assimilated into nurturance). This is what allows us to be able to create and maintain nurturance and happiness.

The stomach dragon memory of enduring without nurturance dims our Spirit's clear/quick perceptions and discriminations for what makes us *happy* and *unhappy* (to help us survive unhappy situations without nurturance that we cannot change or escape).

This 'drag' on the stomach energy circuits that we take on to survive without nurturance or happiness causes us to numb our desire to be nurtured, nurturing or happy. See why there are so many unhappy people in the world? Many are so numb in their stomach circuits that they can't even imagine what might make them happy?

The conscious, elegant solution for stomach energy is to learn to clearly and quickly tune into and discern who and/or what nurtures us. Then we need to take action to connect with whom and/or what is the most nurturing to us physically and emotionally, and learn to disconnect from what is not.

The un-cleared trauma memory that creates stomach issues is about memory of enduring without nurturance and feeling unable or unworthy to make decisions or take actions to fulfill our stomach's Spirit hunger for solution by ingesting what really nurtures us.

Enduring without nurturance creates drag that reduces enzyme production and digestion (which numbs our feelings for happiness, and creates indigestion and unhappiness from inadequate nurturing).

Not being able to choose, ingest and follow our truth about what nurtures and does not nurture us, forces us to defensively endure *without nurturance*. This is a degenerative and unsustainable strategy that will inevitably lead to stomach problems.

5. Anterior Pituitary Spirit Function - Our Master Controller

Our anterior pituitary Spirit Life-force energy is designed to give us the ability to *master our life* with *clear observations* that allow us to direct our energy to coordinate and perform essential actions by delivering the *right dose of the right energy to the right place at the right time*. The anterior pituitary Spirit Life-force energy function provides us with the ability to control, direct and coordinate our destiny effectively and productively in order to *master our life*. It does this by first *observing* and monitoring *what* each organ/gland system needs and *when* it needs it. It then coordinates and organizes the *delivery* of what energy is needed, where and when it's needed, for all aspects of our life and body.

When un-cleared, unconscious trauma memory of either being over-controlled by others, or having no control and direction in our life, is triggered by whatever feels similar in our present life, this memory of anterior pituitary trauma memory reactively projects the old 'drag' onto our ability to consciously master our life and body continuously. Without drag we are able to clearly observe all our organ/gland feelings and coordinate them into our truth and then follow that truth to *master our divine intent.*

149

This drag comes from our trauma memories of having too much or not enough control of our life to learn to productively direct our path from our truth. This causes us to feel as though we are not allowed or capable to master and control our own destiny or that we don't have enough direction to master our life.

These extremes of 'too much or not enough' control traumas in our life create a counter-balancing 'drag' on our anterior pituitary Spirit Life-force energy that is designed to master, control and direct our life.

This drag diminishes our ability to clearly observe quickly and discern what is needed to master, control, direct and coordinate our energy needed to create what we really want when we want and need it. An example of how the dragon creates our present from our past is how the anterior pituitary dragon can become a 'control freak' because energy from traumas of being controlled makes us feel we must be in control to keep from being controlled. (Notice that those who are 'out of control' have a tendency to 'do control' because it is the only thing that gives them a sense of 'being in control'.)

The memory of not feeling safe or able enough to take control and master our life creates a fear of not being able to process, direct and control our life. This causes a hesitating 'drag' on our anterior pituitary energy. And this energy is how we stay clearly connected to our receptors so we may clearly observe what our organ/gland feelings are telling us is needed to coordinate and direct our resources in our moments of power. The key is when we can do it with the right timing so we deliver the right dose at the right time to create what we really want.

Mastery creates effective outcomes by controlling, coordinating, and directing our resources to fulfill our Spirit's needs, dreams and desires in our moments of power. Mastery usually requires consciously getting ahead of old reactive habits of either giving up on controlling our life or over-controlling our life and/or the lives of others. We master our life and body by observing what we need and then directing appropriate control in a timely manner to masterfully deliver *what* is needed *when* it is needed.

The anterior pituitary dragon function memory of not being able to control and direct our life dims our perceptions and discriminations needed to control and direct our powers of observation needed to master our life. Drag allows us to survive defensively by enduring being controlled or having no control over our life. This causes us to numb our Spirit's need to master our own personal lives.

Not feeling or being able to observe and follow our truth to master our destiny by feeling in control of our Life-force energies – forces us to defensively endure feeling we cannot control our life. This is an unsustainable and degenerative consciousness which will inevitably create problems around being able to coordinate and control our life.

6. Liver Spirit Function - Our Transmuter

Our liver Spirit Life-force energy is our organ of *change*. It is designed to give us the ability to *transmute* our energy into what we desire through sufficient focus on creating what we desire. The 'dragon defense' strategy is about *not focusing* on (or not expecting) what we want, in order to *avoid disappointment* from not getting what we want.

Whatever we focus on is what we create from the power of our liver Spirit Life-force energy. Our liver Life-force is needed to create what we want by feeling safe and free to *focus on what we love,* rather than focusing on what we don't have, which creates more of what we don't want.

Disappointment is the 'tell sign' of the *liver trauma dragon* and it comes from not focusing on *what we want* sufficiently to be able to create it, which results in an *expectation of disappointment* (from inadequate ability to create).

This vicious cycle creates disappointment again and again because – **what we focus on is what we create!** So such defensive *negative expectations* prevent us from ever being *able* to think and focus in the way we need to so we can become more *capable* of creating and manifesting what we really desire.

Consequently, *we defeat our Self with our own unconscious fears and unclear thoughts* of negative expectation that, over time, create and fulfill our worst fears: which are about being disappointed!

Consciously using our liver energy to live rather than to age and die requires reversing old habits of enduring and surviving disappointment by giving up on fulfilling our Spirit's desires and expectations.

Transmuting our energy into creating what we desire is a simple basic process of first consciously connecting to our own knowing of what we really want, and then being able to maintain a *steady focus on the actions needed to create and get what we want.* Then, we learn to take those action steps and stay focused on them one at a time, doing the best we can, over a sufficient period to allow them to manifest into our own personal reality.

Our liver Spirit Life-force energy gives us the ability to *rejuvenate our life* by transmuting *what we've got into what we want.* We do this by knowing and focusing on what we want *long enough* to create it while also keeping pace with our changing dynamic times and staying aligned with ourselves and our truth.

Doing this creates rejuvenation and mitigates aging. It does this because it aligns our actions with the dynamic flow of our liver Spirit Life-force energy *so the force of this energy is with us,* which mitigates the resistance or drag that advances aging (created from not allowing our Self to be and express Who we Are as Spirit Life-force energy).

The liver dragon enters the picture when our liver Life-force energy is traumatized and programmed with drag from memories of enduring disappointment from not getting what we really want. This causes drag on our liver perceptions and expressions. Such drag numbs our ability to focus clearly on what we want so we can create it.

Numbing is a basic defensive dragon strategy accomplished by spinning our Life-force energy backward to endure and survive the effects of not being able to effectively create what our Spirit liver energy wants (the Way it was designed to provide when freely perceived and expressed).

The liver dragon's defensive solution to disappointment is to give up on expectation because we can't be disappointed if we don't expect anything.

However, we also must remember that if we can't expect anything we can't create anything either, since the Law of creation is: "What we focus on is what we create!" So, *we must* be able to *expect* something in order to be able to focus on it enough to *create* it.

Triggering old 'memory of disappointment' trauma replays decisions about us giving up on expectation to survive past experiences when we had no choice or power to do anything else. *This 'sets us up' to give up on expectation so we won't be disappointed if we don't expect anything.*

Giving up on expectation diverts us to focus on not getting what we want, which reminds us of our old trauma memory of not getting what we want! This creates a 'relive' of the 'drag' on our liver Life-force energy that *prevents us from creating what we really want.*

The *emotional function of the liver* is designed to provide us with the ability to *transmute through the changes in our life by letting go of what has past, and opening up to what's new* in our present and future.

This ability is needed for us to process the constant changes of our dynamic energetic Reality – with many chances to transmute growth or degeneration – which always is a matter of consciousness in our moments of decision (power) that create either our regenerative or degenerative outcomes.

In other words, our liver provides us with the ability to live by transmuting and rejuvenating our life through constant dynamic changes *if* we learn to focus on what inspires our Spirit to regenerate our life!

The liver energy assists us to change the old into the new. And if the liver circuits are connected, we have no problem figuring out what is needed *that is new and more rejuvenative.* We can judiciously discard what needs to be replaced. Otherwise, we are left *uninspired,* to endure the sadness of not getting what we want, which ages us and prevents the regeneration needed to process our new and changing times.

'Drag' on liver Life-force energy dims our emotional feeling perceptions for discriminating between what can and cannot be transmuted. Being desensitized to disappointment from not getting what we really want strengthens and perpetuates our ability to survive *and endure not getting what we really want.*

This 'drag' on our liver Life-force energy causes us to numb our liver Spirit's desire that gives us the strength to sufficiently focus so we may enact the change we want.

The 'catch phrase' for the liver is: 'transmuting what you've got into what you want.' But the longer version has a little more 'meat' to it which is as follows: "The conscious, elegant solution for liver energy is to transmute 'change' by staying aligned with the flow of our times so we are focusing on *'what we've got'* and how to transmute it into *'what we want.'*" Or, if that's not possible, we will be told by our liver's Spirit Life-force energy (if we are conscious enough to hear it) to find and follow what rejuvenates us in our present and future. Following this truth is what prevents us from aging (the degenerative effect of not living our present truth which shows up by reliving our past memories of not getting what we want).

The elegant solution to this problem is learning to express the liver's Spirit Life-force energy solution, which is to transmute what we've got into what we really want (or to decide 'what we've got' is *not* transmutable and *let it pass* so we can replace it with what *is* transmutable).

7. Lungs Spirit Function - Our Refresher

Our lungs' Spirit Life-force energy is designed to give us the ability to continuously refresh our Life-force energy. It does this by giving us the ability to *breath into our challenges* with feelings of being able to meet them and refresh our strength with Spirit Life-force energy.

Martial arts have always utilized breathing to give power to performances. This is because most challenges *must ideally be met in the moment* by 'breathing in' our primary source of power called 'prana.' Prana immediately empowers our physical and emotional actions with the strength to enact our elegant solutions in our moments of power.

Such solutions require us to be conscious enough in the moment of our breathing to keep ahead of old reactive unconscious habits of holding our breath – (since not breathing severely stifles our Spirit Life-force energy flow that is needed to provide our elegant solutions.)

There are all different types of 'breath holding.' Of course, the most serious one is when we stop breathing completely which inevitably results in not only a stifling of Spirit Life-force, but is quickly followed by death! And then there is the kind where we hyper-ventilate because we have taken in more oxygen than we need – plus everything else 'in between' in the way of holding our breath. Again, it's about 'dosing and timing' and being very conscious about what kind of breathing we do and what those results are.

Prana is the breath of Life-force energy that allows us to perform most effectively in all we do well. We can survive without water, food and shelter for limited periods of time – but without our Spirit's breath of 'prana' Life-force energy to help maintain our homeostasis, we are dead within minutes!

Our breath is our primary moment-to-moment source of here-and-now Life-force prana energy – and our lungs are the primary processor of this prana energy! To maximize our power from the prana breath it must be full, continuous, rhythmic breathing in perfect alignment with the feelings of our emotional flow of whatever we are experiencing in our life – we must breathe with our body's flow of feelings.

Proper breathing keeps pranic Life-force energy moving through our body to energize and detoxify our system. This exchange removes the toxic 'drag' from our circuits when we breathe in long, slow, deep continuous diaphragmatic breaths (without holds) that *flow in a connected way with what we see and feel.*

Our breath is designed to provide us with the energy we need to successfully meet our most demanding and challenging moments in life. But this all depends on whether or not *we are breathing correctly.* We do this by practicing 'breathing into' our challenging moments with proper flow. A great example of this is the way an opera singer regulates her timing to *precisely align with the Laws of energy* (in the realm of sound/music).

We need to align our behavioral performances with how our Spirit Life-force aligns with the Law/Ways of energy to best perform what is needed to create our goal – when the power of these Laws is aligned with us to meet and match our challenges. How well we learn to do this is revealed by how we show up in our moments of power as being either effective or ineffective at *productively meeting our challenges.*

The *lung dragon* enters the picture when our lung Spirit Life-force energy is *traumatized* (programmed or conditioned) into holding our breath to stifle our pain to 'not feel' whatever 'bad' we were feeling. The lung dragon's solution to such traumas of 'feeling stifled' is to *learn to better endure and survive being stifled by holding our breath.* This then becomes an *unconscious reactive memory pattern* (habit) that gets triggered and projected wherever possible – until we become conscious enough of it to *get ahead of it* in our moments of power.

Holding our breath stops us from feeling (i.e. like how we hold our breath when we enter cold water to not feel the cold so much). When there is a drag on our lung Spirit Life-force energy, this drag shows up emotionally as 'not feeling and following our natural breath to meet and match our challenges.'

What holding our breath does is to disconnect us from our truth and true feelings (the very things that give us our personal power), which causes us to not be able to meet our challenges. This is *why we hold our breath* when we get in cold water – so we don't have to *feel the cold water!*

By holding our breath or by shallow breathing, we *shut off our feelings* (so we *supposedly* don't have to deal with them) and then continue to play the defensive game for which the lung dragon is famous.

Drag numbs our ability to breathe into our challenges to meet them most effectively, but provides a good short-term defensive strategy for 'not feeling' pain or discomfort. But the strategy of not breathing (as an unconscious habit pattern for dealing with challenges) spins our Life-force energy backward, to defensively endure and survive the effects of not breathing into our challenges immediately to solve them in the 'here and now.'

The *emotional function of our lungs* is to breathe into our challenges and consciously align with our Spirit Life-force energy powers to immediately and continuously *refresh* our Life-force energy. Without the ability to *spontaneously breathe into and through our challenges* in our moments of power, we suffer *great losses in our personal ability* when we need our strength the most to be productive.

Unconscious habits of *not breathing deeply enough to really feel what we are feeling* disconnects us from our lungs' Spirit Life-force energy to endure chronic issues without meeting the challenges needed to refresh us. This is an unsustainable, degenerative strategy and will inevitably lead to lung problems.

8. Sex Organs Spirit Function - Our Connectors

Our sex organs' Spirit Life-force energy gives us the ability to connect with others on four different levels of energy (physical, emotional, mental and Spirit Life force energy). When all of these energy levels *connect in safety, Love and harmony* with the true essence of Who we really are as Spirit, this opens up how we think, talk and *connect with our Self and others.* When we do this on all levels spontaneously we are more able to connect more completely with our Self by *feeling worthy of love being true to our Self.*

When we are able to feel safe being vulnerable, we can open up clearly on an emotional level and reveal our true feelings so they flow through our organ/gland energy circuits spontaneously and appropriately.

We do this by first feeling safe and secure in knowing and connecting with our truth and being able to perform it spontaneously in a respectable way that creates and maintains real harmony and fulfillment to keep our relationships securely connected with real Love.

How we react and respond in our processing of these moments of power will determine how successful we are at interacting personally with others (measured by what is sustainable and regenerative). It's all about how we perform mentally, emotionally and physically (intimately) in our relationships.

Relationships require us to consciously stay 'ahead of' (and out of) *triggered reactions* from associations with *unconscious trauma memory* of dysfunctional relationships that separate and disconnect us so we 'feel incapable and unworthy' of having a successful relationship. (Feeling unworthy makes us look and/or feel and act more unworthy, so we tend to attract others who are controlled by this same dragon energy (which I refer to as a match made in hell!)

I tell my clients that *God gives us relationships in case we don't go to therapy!* This is true because relationships will *push all our buttons* (triggers) because they are so *up close and personal* (the way they need to be to feel and be real). But we can only *keep this real intimate connection* if we can *keep it real* and *stay ahead of our triggered reactions* consciously. This allows us to make better energetic choices quicker that work things out smoother and more often in our relationships.

The sex organ dragon's ways are ***not*** about supporting our Spirit agenda *to be and feel safe connecting and feeling worthy of real Love in relationships.* The sex organ dragons are born from the *memory of separation and disconnection trauma.* So, by their very nature, dragons do not expect their relationships to feel safe or be worthy or interested in real love. Real love would mean *putting others' best interests first,* and the dragon energy is not designed to do that because it is a *self interested survival mechanism.* So having a 'safe connection' that feels trust 'worthy' with a dragon is not imaginable to the dragon because it contradicts the energetic Reality that defines the dragon's nature.

If you can't trust, you can't connect – and if you can't connect, then you can't have a 'real' relationship!

Safe connections come from being and feeling sufficiently safe enough to open up and allow a real connection to happen. How else could this ever happen? It has to be a real connection with our Spirit to feel and be real! Dragons are not 'who we are.' They are 'who we are not' – or what I call – the *'not you.'*

Engaging with dragon energy in relationships only makes things worse! It strengthens and justifies the *'not you,'* which is not what our Spirit is interested in doing *if and when* it has the power as well as the freedom to make Spirit oriented decisions in our relationships. Withdrawing from a 'dragon relationship' only confirms the dragons' most core belief – which I call 'dragon trust', which is: "You can never trust anybody about anything…ever!" This is why many people 'can't find love again' after a failed relationship. Their dragon realizes what is at stake to make the connection real and successful, and if it is 'in charge', it will find a trillion reasons not to 'ever trust anybody ever again' even though the truth is we is that we can't have the relationship we want without worthy trust.

Any connected relationship relies on both parties ability to trust and connect. The sex organ dragon only trusts learning to endure and survive. It does this by *'living' in separation and disconnection* but acting like it is connecting *without really connecting.* But this is not really **living!** This is why *dragons feel like relationships are hopeless,* because if you *must trust* but you *can't trust* – they *are* hopeless! And as unsafe as this defensive strategy is, it is the dragons' *only strategy available for having a relationship.*

Engaging with dragon energy is always a trap because *without trust being possible,* we could never feel safe having a trustworthy relationship. If our dragon consciously holds this 'unsafe' attitude and energy, this ensures that *nobody who is fully conscious will ever trust us to be a safe connection for them.* This almost guarantees that we will be without real connections for our entire lives. And this is sad to me because from observing thousands of clients, I have come to believe that our quest for real *connection in our relationships* may be *our primary human drive.*

Being without personal connections continuously creates chronic *apathy.* This apathy comes from not feeling safe and worthy of Love. But once we feel safe and worthy of love within our Self, it allows for us to open up and have relationships with other loving enlightened Spirits which eliminates our apathy!

Finding and connecting with others who are capable and worthy of real connections allows us to regenerate our life and body – rather than degenerate in relationships that never give us what we want.

If we don't feel safe and worthy of love within our Self, we can never show up being Who we really are! And if we can't show up being Who We Are, any relationship we have will be with 'who we are not' and then someday we'll wake up and tell our 'partner': *"You don't even know Who I Am!"* (And the answer is: "Of course not, because since you never really showed up – *how could I really know Who You Are?"*).

Living *without connections* – while connection is a primary innate desire and need for us – obviously creates a serious *connection problem*. This is especially true if most of our relationship experiences with human connections were *never worthy of trust* – since trust is the essential ingredient to ever having and maintaining any *real relationship connections!*

Connecting with others in a regenerative manner first requires that we *feel safe and worthy of love within our Self* and have sufficient consciousness to be able to discern between those who are capable of maintaining continuous *loving and enlightening connections* – and those who maintain continuous *unloving and unenlightened disconnections.* These *disconnections* cover up their real truth with *pretense* and *reactivity* and this is why they end up *separating and disconnecting* in their relationships.

Our sex organs' Spirit Life-force energy is designed to give us the ability to *attract and create Life-force* energy through connections that achieve their potential productive results or reproduction (as in biological math, where 1+1=3).

Sex organ energy is needed to maintain the species as well as to *inspire, energize and regenerate* the health of our entire life and body. Sexual stimulation creates surges of electrical energy throughout the body that can climax in spontaneous *organ spasms* that flush out and release *static electrical charges of drag* on our organ/gland energy circuits. Orgasm might in some ways be considered 'God's health plan' for helping to clear the drag on our organ/gland Life-force energy circuits!

The *sex organ dragon* enters the picture when our sex organ Life-force energy is *traumatized* and programmed by drag with trauma memories of *feeling separated and disconnected from others who feel* like they *do not have our best interests in mind.* So the sex organ dragon enters when we *feel this disconnection from others* to protect us by *connecting without really connecting* with others when forced to connect with those who don't feel safe. This is why we end up not feeling *safe enough* to ever really *open up enough to be real enough* to ever have a *real connected relationship that feels like it's 'enough.'*

This causes us to unconsciously and reactively go on the *defensive* by separating and disconnecting, while we learn to *'connect without really connecting'* in any real way *with anyone.* We take on the

159

sex organ dragon which gives us the 'drag' on our Life-force needed to *separate and disconnect from our true Spirit Self.* This is why the dragon will end up spending so much energy *acting like it is being real **without being real*** (which is an energetically degenerative practice).

Defensive strategies always spin our energy backward, which disconnects us from our Self and causes us to *not feel like we are able* to really connect with others. But our energy needs to go backward to operate defensively to better endure and *survive the effects of being in disconnected,* untrustworthy relationships. Being in these negative relationships actually 'subtracts' our Life-force energy from us and makes our life a drag – instead of 'multiplying' our Life-force energy to make our life fulfilling and inspiring!

If the sexual organs' Spirit Life-force energy is taken over by the dragon, the dragon's need for *disconnection* will soon cause feelings of *apathy* to set in because that is what separation and disconnection from true Self connections with meaningful trustworthy relationships feels like.

Un-cleared *trauma memory of disconnection* from feeling unsafe and being unable to connect, attract and fulfill our desires for connection causes us to *disconnect from ourselves.* Then that naturally creates a tendency in us to unconsciously do what we've always done – which is to disconnect from others to defensively avoid re-experiencing unsafe connection trauma.

The dark brilliance of the sex organ dragon's solution is to just have *more unreal connections* 'behind the scenes,' to make up for our *lack of real connections* and fulfillment from our primary *relationships.* And then, the dragon *covers the truth of our disconnections* while defensively counterbalancing that emptiness by creating the 'illusion of connection' for others to see. Either way, the dragon thinks that in order for it to survive, it must endure and survive disconnection in relationships since it cannot trust.

The truth is, that in order 'to survive' we may have 'to endure' certain things. But *fulfillment is not about the ways of survival.* We reach a point in our personal evolution where, *if* we really do need to be 'in defense' to feel safe we should *not* be there or with that person! But if it really is safe to be with someone, *then* we should *not be 'in defense'* because it destroys the connection we need to fulfill us.

In order to connect with others, we have to be able to connect with our true Self *first,* because we cannot connect with anyone or anything else *any better* than we are connected to our true Self (twenty-three organ/gland feelings – energy systems). Without this connection with our Self, we automatically connect with others through our *'not you,'* so we have a 'not you connection' with them – not a *real connection* with our *'Real You'!* So it will not feel like a *real* connection to us either! We could call it a "not relationship," because it will feel like we are *not* really having a relationship (that is real)!

The *Spirit function of the sex organs* is designed to discern *worthy connections* by clearly and quickly sensing who feels *emotionally safe* and noticing the differences between who feels safe and real enough to open up to and really connect with, and who does not (because they don't feel safe and/or believable as far as having our best interests in mind).

Drag on our sex organs Spirit Life-force energy (defense) diminishes our ability to feel inspired by our emotional feelings of attraction, connection and creation. In other words, our Spirit is only designed to connect with *those who are capable of having 'our Spirit's best interest' in mind.* Otherwise, we are playing defense, and there are *no points for defense!*

The 'drag' on our sex organ energy that we 'take on' to survive 'not connecting' causes us to *numb or pervert our natural desire to really connect.*

The conscious, elegant solution for the sex organ energy is to learn to choose safe, respectful, loving, responsible people who can really stay connected to us on the level of our Spirit's Ways. This means not accepting anything less than real connections, *otherwise* that passive 'acceptance' becomes the primary reinforcer, enabler and maintainer of the very problem that is out of alignment with our Spirit. In this case, it would be the dragon 'player' philosophy that is about maintaining an unreal, disconnected relationship while pretending to them that it is *more than that.*

The un-cleared trauma memories that create sex organ issues are often related to not feeling *safe being real* and then not feeling *accepted being real.* This becomes very confusing when we must figure out *who is real* by observing clearly who really loves and accepts the Real You!

Following our sex organ Spirit's Ways of energy means only *connecting with those who we feel safe being vulnerable with* and who continue to show up and verify by their deeds that they have our *best interests in mind.* This is the only thing that really works productively in our relationships! Otherwise, we can't really connect because we don't feel safe to open up and connect.

9. Bones and Muscles Spirit Function - Our Responders

The bones and muscles issues have to do with *movement* to either *approach or avoid* what we want and don't want. We do this so we can *get closer* to what we want and *further away* from what we don't want. Bone and muscle energy is designed to sense, feel, and move away from what causes *pain,* and toward what *inspires and fulfills* our Spirit's desires. In order to *stop our inclination to move* away or leave; the body needs *toxic drag* on our bones and muscles (anything from junk food to prescription medication) to *'numb the pain' of 'not moving' away from painful situations or toward what our Spirit wants.*

Bone and muscle Spirit Life-force energy unconsciously conditions and programs us to endure and survive *present* painful situations that trigger us to *think* we cannot change or escape them. This energy originated from the *trauma memory* of having to endure and survive *past painful situations that we could not change or escape.*

The bones and muscles dragon encourages us to just *endure pain* with enough 'drag' to *not respond* with locomotion in order to avoid pain. And when we are no longer inspired to *move* toward (approach) our Spirit's desires; this drag continues in us to resist using our bones and muscles to move as they are designed to do. When this happens, we experience *stiffening* that further *limits our ability to move freely.* This stiff body language reflects a lack of a clear *movement connection* with our true Spirit Self.

Having 'drag' on bone and muscle Spirit Life-force energy is often observed in the proud *martyr,* when the *'dragon expresses its pride'* over its considerable ability to endure painful situations by saying things like, *"It's not that bad compared to what I've endured! I can handle whatever it is! I've endured worse."*

The bone and muscle Spirit Life-force energy is about using our physical tools – body, bones and muscles – that perform our everyday *movements* as they also provide amply 'tells' for other aspects of our life. Every *body part* is a metaphor that is conceptually related to a *function*. For example, our *hands* may reflect how we *handle* things; our *eyes*, how we *see* things; our *heart*, how we *love*.

Our mind's memory, ideas, concepts, associations and traumas around 'movement' unconsciously foretell how we will *think and 'conceptualize' how we can direct our movements* to either *align or misalign* with how we really *feel emotionally*. This creates some very 'telling' body language that can either give us *points,* or *penalties –* which determines our *ability* or *inability* to move and perform with innate *believability*.

Flexibility in our lives and bodies requires sufficient conscious-ness to process and flow with *being here now* consistently in order to 'stay ahead of' triggered reactive projections of unconscious memory and old habits of drag. It is about either being directed in our 'moments of decision' to *move or not move* now, as we did *then* in our memory. But in our past unconscious triggered memory, 'then' we had no per-sonal power. This is another example of how past memory *projects old 'reruns' as they resurrect old 'relive's of when we had no choice* (as if it were true *now*).

So only our own consciousness for Reality 'here and now' can give us a clear conscious view and choice in our 'moments of power' to be able to act ahead of the *curve* (created by our *reactive moments*), to give us access to our true Spirit Life-force power. *Not moving* with our *Spirit's truth* requires having a drag on our Spirit's response to move *toward* our divine intent and *away* from painful situations.

Clear responsive movements require sufficient consciousness in the present moment to clearly perceive quickly what we do want and what we don't want – to be able to initiate *movement* toward what we want and away from what we don't want. Otherwise, if we uncon-sciously buy into what we don't want, by default we reinforce, enable and maintain what we don't want. This misaligns with our Spirit's truth, and expresses this misalignment in an 'unbelievable' body language that sacrifices our grace and beauty whole holding us hostage to pain.

The *bone and muscle* dragon enters the picture when we take on drag on our bone and muscle Life-force energy flow from triggers unconsciously associated with trauma memories of feelings and ideas from when it was 'not safe to move' *toward* what we wanted or *away from* what we didn't want. When this was the case, we felt we had to *take on drag to stop us from responding to our pains and desires with locomotion* and movement toward what we want and away from what we don't want.

Such reactive memories and behavior patterns persist unconsciously, and when they are triggered and repeatedly acted out in our present life, we maintain bone and muscle drag on our Spirit Life-force energy flow to perform with attractive and believable movement!

The *bone and muscle dragon's solution* for dealing with pain is to *numb it and endure it,* which adds to our *feeling unsafe and unable to move* away from pain (or toward what we want); so the dragon solution is to *endure and/or survive the pain of not* moving away from painful situations or toward desirable ones.

Conscious awareness of the drag that numbs our ability to notice pain and respond to it appropriately is essential. Our bone and muscle Spirit Life-force energy would naturally, spontaneously, and automatically move if we didn't have conscious or unconscious drag on it. This is why triggered memory of drag creates *hesitation* in our actions and takes personal power from our performances.

Drag, however does provide a great defense that allows us to endure painful situations by spinning our energy backward to numb our senses and survive painful situations when no hope exists for a solution.

The emotional function of our bones and muscles allows us to discern our feelings for when, where, and how to move and in what direction to approach the positive or avoid the negative painful situations. This is our approach/avoidance movement mechanism.

At our Spirit level we have the natural Life-force ability to flow in our responses that align with our true feelings toward what feels good and away from what does not. Drag on bone and muscle Spirit Life-force energy diminishes our sensitivity to our emotional feelings for what is painful and what is inspiring, which then causes us to endure what we don't want and ignore what we do want.

The 'drag' on bone and muscle Spirit Life-force energy that we take on to endure not moving causes us to feel disabled and unable to do what we need to do.

The conscious, elegant solution for the bone and muscle Spirit Life-force energy is to perceive the subtle aspects of painful situations *long before* we are in them up to our ears; and if we are already in them, to be willing and able to *leave them quickly.*

The un-cleared *reactive trauma memory* creating bone and muscle issues is *feeling that we could not move toward or away from what we did or didn't want.* Instead we had to physically and emotionally not respond truthfully while we endure painful situations that in the *past* we couldn't change or escape.

Not noticing and following our bone and muscle Spirit Life-force energy responses to move us away from what we don't want and toward what we do want, clearly, quickly and appropriately, is (over time) a degenerative strategy that will inevitably manifest as movement issues and bone and muscle problems.

10. Thyroid Spirit Function - Our Corrector

Our thyroid Spirit Life-force energy gives us the ability to *take corrective action* toward whatever provokes *anxiety* from things *not* being 'right' or 'aligned' with justice for our Spirit. This is when and how anxiety is a 'good thing' and *why it needs to be noticed* when we are 'Spirit moved' in this way!

Thyroid Spirit energy is designed to provide us with instant energy (in the form of anxiety) to take action to correct injustices or indignities to our Spirit. Injustice to our Spirit Self creates feelings of *anxiety* to *energize our actions* to correct injustices in our life and body and return to a feeling of *balanced justice.*

Expressing our anxiety by *taking action* to correct what doesn't 'feel right' or feels like an *injustice,* uses our thyroid energy ability to *make right* what is *not right* for us. This requires consciously *getting ahead of our old familiar habits of drag* (in our moments of power/ decision) so we may consciously allow our actions to do *now* what we couldn't (or wouldn't) do then to correct personal injustices.

Doing this requires us to first be able to instantly and consciously *perceive personal injustices* or things of danger, and then we must be able to *express our provoked anxiety* so we correct the problem by *creating* what is right by virtue of our behavior *aligning* with the regenerative Ways/Laws of energy.

Correcting what is 'not right' requires sufficient consciousness to be able to quickly have clear spontaneous *perceptions* and take appropriate effective *action* consistently and immediately by being able to see and articulate 'what is not right' and what to do to 'make it right.'

The ability to *articulate effectively* helps immensely, especially if we can do it *spontaneously* in less than 1.1 second – which is our 'moment of power' where we have maximum power to be *believable and effective*. This is the *only thing that works* very effectively, consistently, and also sells movie tickets – because doing it this quickly and clearly defines what 'being believable' means!

The *thyroid dragon* enters the picture when our *present experiences* trigger old trauma memory associations of 'drag' on justice to our Spirit – by *not taking actions* to claim our own personal justice.

This causes us to think and *feel we cannot get or expect 'personal justice'* for what is right for us, so "We just shouldn't think about it." Such drag perpetuates itself and numbs our ability to even *notice* what feels 'right and just,' because we are too busy suppressing/numbing or overreacting to our injustices.

Our *reactive defensive numbing* creates even *more* personal injustice, which justifies even more drag to allow us to be able to endure and survive even more personal injustice. The thyroid dragon solution to traumas of personal injustice is to learn better to endure and survive injustice *without notice or correction*.

Our Spirit always notices injustice, on some level of consciousness. 'Not noticing' is a great defensive 'prison strategy.' But the only real question is: "How long do you want to stay in prison?" Because *enduring injustice daily is a prison* that will cost us dearly!

If our thyroid Spirit Life-force energy has been conditioned and directed by reactive, un-cleared trauma/dragon memory to unconsciously over accept injustices in our life – then we will *fear taking just action to correct our injustices.* This behavior will continue to reinforce, enable and maintain our own personal injustice. Do you see the trap?

This trap is a drag on our ability to first perceive personal injustice and then to take action to correct it! 'Not noticing' and 'not showing-up' forces us to internalize our anxieties by doing nothing about the injustice to our Self. This invites and leaves us open to further injustices from those delivering it and will lead to continuous *free floating anxiety.*

As the old saying goes (again), *"If we don't stand for something, we could fall for anything!"* If we stand up for what is right for us (and learn to do it clearly, quickly and appropriately), we get to *see who cares* about us by how they act in term of what is right for us, so we feel honored by others who support our right to expect to be treated right in terms of personal justice.

*By not taking actio*n to correct our injustices, we accept, enable and maintain our injustices – by internalizing the anxiety feelings of not expressing the energy that empowers us to protect our present and future from living in personal injustice.

When we suppress this energy, it creates a drag on our metabolic functions and on our body's ability to give us energy for daily life – while also contributing to hypothyroid or hyperthyroid problems: being either underactive or overactive.

The emotional function of the thyroid gives us the ability to perceive and take action directed from feelings of personal injustice when such things come up. For instance, if we feel that something is *not fair* – we will actually say something like "This isn't fair!" instead of saying and doing nothing about the personal injustices in our lives.

You might be surprised to know how many people do not feel like they can ever say anything about the personal injustices in their lives. This is usually because they have been trained in these situations to be 'longsuffering', 'love their neighbor', 'be kind', etcetera (which is very convenient programming for the dragon if everyone stays 'unreal' about how they really feel about personal injustices).

Having a drag on thyroid Spirit Life-force energy diminishes our feeling for what is 'right' and 'wrong' for us. This then results in enduring what is wrong for us *without taking any effective action to correct what is wrong and make it right* so that we may create a new life story about our personal justice.

However, not saying anything about personal injustices – goes against Spirit promptings. In other words, we have been designed with the ability to *emotionally feel personal injustices* (through anxiety) and then use that energy to spontaneously take *appropriate corrective action as soon as possible.*

The 'drag' on thyroid energy that we take on to endure not correcting what's not right for us, over time causes us to feel that we don't deserve what is right for us and further encourages us to not notice the personal injustices in our life from our Spirit's point of view. Our conscious Spirit solution for the thyroid energy is to first perceive the subtle aspects of what is right and wrong for us, clearly and quickly – and then take action to correct it.

The un-cleared trauma/memory that creates thyroid issues is the feeling of having to endure personal injustice and feeling we cannot change or escape our situation.

Not following our thyroid Spirit truth to correct injustice is degenerative. If you don't correct injustice, then you put up with it. If you put up with it you are going to reinforce, enable and maintain injustice which attracts injustice and is therefore not a sustainable, regenerative strategy. It will inevitably lead to more personal injustice and then to the denser energy of physical thyroid problems.

11. Veins and Arteries Spirit Function - Our Circulator

The Spirit Life-force energy of our veins and arteries gives us the feeling and ability to *circulate and participate in the games of life by feeling* free of restriction to flow with our Spirit Life-force energy. The manifestation of this feeling energy in our body is our *veins and arteries* circulating our blood/Life-force energy freely to distribute and deliver nurturance to all our organs, glands and cells.

This requires us to be conscious – *in or before the moment of deciding – to stay ahead* of old familiar habits of enduring restrictions by ignoring our Spirit's desire to *circulate and participate unrestricted.*

Circulation and participation in the games of life requires sufficient consciousness to make new decisions in or before the moments that reactively *trigger our unconscious habits of automatic restriction* of our Spirit's *spontaneous response to circulate and participate* in what life offers.

The *veins and arteries dragon* enters the picture when our veins and arteries' Spirit Life-force energy is *traumatized* by whatever causes us to *feel restricted* from flowing freely with our Spirit to participate in the games of life. This memory of restricting our circulation and participation becomes an old habit that creates new memory that conditions us even more with drag on feeling free to circulate and participate. This makes freely circulating and participating feel unfamiliar and uncomfortable. Consequently, we continue to reinforce, enable and maintain *restrictions on our Self* that make us more able to e*ndure restricted circulation* and less able to effectively *participate in the games of life*.

'Drag' on Spirit Life-force numbs our ability to even notice where, when and how we are making decisions that restrict ourselves from circulating and participating in the games of life. This drag on our energy-motion will eventually manifest physically in our veins and arteries as actual mass and matter that restrict our circulation, flow and distribution of nutrients to our life and body through our blood vessels.

This restricted behavior of *drag on circulating and participating* provides defensive numbing by spinning our energy backward defensively. Numbing our feelings enables us to endure and survive our restrictions. Until these feelings are numbed, the subtle prompting to circulate and 'dance' in the games of life can become quite nagging to the dragon. So, the more numb these feelings become, the easier it gets to ignore the message of Spirit Life-force to the veins and arteries on a 'short term' level. However, long term this restrictive behavior contributes to high blood pressure and varicose veins.

The veins and arteries dragon solution to traumas of feeling restricted is to learn how to better *numb, endure and survive restriction*, and then rationalize it so we *don't really notice it.* However, our Spirit always notices it, consciously or subconsciously– even if our Spirit does not have the consciousness to give us the power to do anything about it! So again, this is a great prison strategy, but the real question is, "How long do you want to *stay in a prison of restrictions* on circulating and participating in your life?"

The *emotional function of the veins and arteries* gives us the ability to consciously feel the differences between *feeling free to circulate, participate and communicate,* versus feeling r*estricted, isolated and resentful.* In other words, our Spirit's emotional feelings are designed *to flow freely, to circulate, connect and communicate as so inclined.*

When we allow a drag/restriction on our veins and arteries' Spirit Life-force energy to take over our way of life, it creates a v*icious declining cycle* that further diminishes our emotional ability to consciously *even feel the restriction. This causes us to further limit our circulation and participation, which results in making* more decisions and actions that further restrict us.

The drag on our veins and arteries' Spirit Life-force energy that we take on to endure further restriction causes us to feel that we don't want to circulate or participate. And as time goes on, that becomes the attitude of our dragon's unconscious philosophy, which then directs our decisions and actions.

The elegant Spirit solution for our veins and arteries energy is to be conscious in our moments of power of our subtle decisions and actions that restrict us with time-warps of memory that disconnect us from our power to make a different decision about circulating and participating here and now.

The un-cleared trauma memories over time that create vein and artery issues leave us with a persistent feeling that we have to endure restrictions while feeling there is no way out; or, that we could never change or escape the *real* or even the *unreal* restrictions.

Perceiving and following our veins and arteries' Spirit truth so we can stay ahead of our unconscious programming for restricting our circulation and participation, *prevents* degeneration by creating regeneration from making decisions to circulate and participate.

Enduring restriction is an unsustainable, defensive strategy that further restricts our circulation, which will inevitably create circulation (resulting in vein and artery) problems in our body as well as participation difficulties in the various aspects of our life.

12. Brain and Nervous System Spirit Function - Our Simplifier

Our brain and nervous system Spirit Life-force energy represents our 'power lines' (nerves) that allow all other powers to communicate, integrate and express *simplification, before complication takes over*. This is only possible because we are equipped with an 'organized' electrical nervous system that provides continuous bioelectrical connection, flow and communication between all our organ/gland energy systems and functions when it is directed by our Spirit. If not, it will be unconsciously controlled and directed by our dragons with drag here and there creating *static* on connections and flow of energy. See the problem?

Spirit-directed and motivated electrical nervous system Life-force energy flows spontaneously with perfect timing (when without drag/ static) that aligns with the Laws of energy and naturally sequences our challenges to best meet our demands by just 'tuning in' to what our nervous system is telling us.

This is done by consciously 'tuning in' to our nervous system feelings of electrical energy that connects to all our organ/gland perceptions and expressions needed to fulfill whatever our life and body needs, when, where and how it is needed. When allowed to, this natural spontaneous nervous system function simplifies our life before complications happen by being ahead of the curve to avoid them.

This is our electrical energy grid system that communicates all our organ/gland Life-force energy functions of perceptions and expressions. The brain is our Life-force energy organizer – our internal 'day timer.' It allows us to organize and direct our life in a timely manner by directing our electrical energy flow to the right place at the right time. This energy flow is needed to *perceive record, transmit and express* all our conscious and unconscious Life-force energy thoughts, feelings and actions – mentally, emotionally and physically.

This requires consciously understanding and getting ahead of old familiar reactive habits of not noticing and enduring and enabling complications while ignoring our Spirit's simple Ways. Spirit's Ways of being clear quick and appropriate enable us to make decisions and take actions that align with solutions that 'simplify our reality,' so we may avoid later unnecessary confusions and complications.

The brain and nervous system dragon enters the picture when our brain and nervous system Life-force energy gets programmed and conditioned by trauma memories of having to endure and survive continuous confusions and complications without order, without an end or without solutions.

This trauma programming creates drag on the electrical energy flow (expression) of our true feelings. The expression of how we really feel will simplify our life by avoiding later complications *if* we confront and clear the static now – rather than spinning our brain and nervous system energy backward while avoiding the truth. These kinds of defensive choices are inspired by an unconscious, reactive drag to suppress our truth which results inevitably in having to endure the resulting confusions and complications.

When this memory of enduring the confusions and complications is unconsciously triggered, it can reactively take over our brain and nervous system with the memory of having to live in confusion and complications that we couldn't figure out how to change or escape (so we could never *simplify* our life's situation of complicated confusions).

Defensive strategies ignore and endure our complicated confusions and require us to take on even more 'drag' (black body mass) to resist and numb our nervous system from feeling our confusions without acting to simplify our complications. We accomplish defensive homeostasis by counterbalancing our Spirits' truth with drag on our perceptions and expressions of our most authentic thoughts and feelings concerning the complications – with plenty of distractions that disable us from doing what we must do to simplify our life.

This drag creates pressure and feelings of nervousness that arise from excess energy/pressure in our nervous system. This makes us more reactive and may cause bursting, splitting headaches. These are often accompanied by a 'fog of confusion' that makes life seem very complicated and difficult because we can't clearly and quickly connect the dots and act on them. We feel like we can't get anything done because our nervous system is too jammed with drag on our circuits of Life-force energy flow or power!

Such drag numbs our ability to even notice the confusions and complications in our life, which is the brain and nervous system dragon's defensive strategy of numbing our perceptions and then enduring the confusions and complications that result from not doing what we need to in the moment we notice. Not noticing our complications spins our energy backward into defense, to better endure and survive what we think we cannot change or escape because we cannot imagine it – so from this view point, it is hopeless!

Our Spirit (consciously or subconsciously) always notices our truth, so not noticing is a great prison strategy but the real question is, "How long do we want to stay in the prison of enduring confusions and complications?" Playing defense means playing without the ball (our truth). This also means we can't make any points without revealing our truth – so we end up not getting any points by playing defense!

The emotional function of the brain and nervous system is designed to clearly, immediately and appropriately discriminate between the feelings of simplicity and those nervous feelings of confusions and complications. In other words, we are designed with the emotional ability to feel certain directives from our Spirit that can guide and direct our path if we recognize and follow them quickly.

Triggered old memories of *enduring confusions* create drag on our brain and nervous system Life-force energy flow if our consciousness is unable to stay ahead of the unconscious curve. Living behind the curve diminishes our emotional sensitivity to *feel* what we need to feel, in order to *do (which is to create and promote simplicity by learning to consciously live 'ahead of the curve')*. We can then eliminate our confusions and complications by learning to consistently express our truth clearly, quickly and appropriately to keep from feeling the nervous system pressure that would result from not doing this.

The 'drag' on our brain and nervous system Spirit Life-force energy that we take on to endure our confusions and complications causes us to feel like giving up on ever having simplicity in our life.

The conscious, elegant solution for the brain and nervous system energy is to consciously use our Spirit's ability to be clear and quick enough to perceive and take actions that discern the differences between doing what creates simplicity versus doing what creates confusions and complications.

In summary, the un-cleared trauma memories that create brain and nervous system issues are a history of having to endure confusions and complications. When this memory is reactivated of 'what we could not change or escape *then,*' we must be conscious enough to choose to solve life's 'brain game' proactively in the moment by learning to recognize, express and act on the ways we can simplify our lives.

Connecting with and following our brain and nervous system's Spirit truth by making decisions for energetic simplicity that avoid confusions and complications *is* regenerative because we clarify and organize to resolve degenerative confusions and their complications *before we create them.* Not 'showing up' to do this consistently in the moment – will inevitably lead to brain and nervous system problems.

13. Adrenals Spirit Function - Our 'Empowerer'

Our adrenal Spirit Life-force energy gives us the capacity to respond to life's pressures by being able to match them with *equal and opposite pressures* by using our adrenal power to confront and resolve conflicts.

Spirit Ways are direct and fair so they allow our Spirit to feel personal pride by just having the courage to 'show up' being Who (Spirit) we really are.

Performing adrenal power comes from first having sufficient courage to confront and meet the pressure of opposition with the *equal and opposite pressure* of our position (op-position). We do this by standing up for ourselves in the heat of conflict with clear concepts that reflect and articulate our position effectively in a believable manner without being *overpowering*. This Way of doing things also prevents us from being overpowered by opposing forces.

The adrenal dragon enters the picture when our adrenal Life-force energy is programmed and conditioned with drag from trauma memories of having to endure and survive feeling and being overpowered by our world and circumstances around us, preventing us from learning, knowing and effectively mastering our own personal power.

If our adrenal Spirit Life-force energy gets programmed and conditioned by trauma memory of 'drag' on our personal power, it creates a feeling of shame from the feeling of being overpowered and having no power. Such triggers causes us to unconsciously associate, project and reactivate past memory of 'drag' on our adrenal Spirit Life-force energy to perform under pressure in our present – just like we were programmed and conditioned to do in our past when we felt we had no power.

This creates a feeling of fatigue from disempowerment, which physically drains our energy and makes us feel incapable of dealing with any kind of pressure. So we remain unaware of the possibility of making choices that meet pressure with equal and opposite pressure (which was not perceived as being possible in our past).

But in the present, meeting our pressures with equal and opposite pressure may now provide the only pathway to create our elegant solutions to effectively process our pressure-charged situations quickly and appropriately. It just takes courage, consciousness and a script for how to do it in the kind of productive manner that allows us to live and be real in our present moments.

Adrenal drag holds back our primary energy/power system that gives us energy for our own personal empowerment that is needed to counter life's pressures that we face daily in our lives. Plus, this drag lessens our ability to even notice where, when and how we unconsciously give up on our own personal power, without a second thought, by just following our old dysfunctional and degenerative habits.

Not noticing the drag on our personal power, is part of our adrenal dragon's defensive strategy of numbing our perceptions of *where, when and how we lose or give away our power.* Adrenal drag spins our Life-force power backward so we can better endure and survive without it. This causes us to repeat *now* what we 'had to' do *then* in the past when we had 'no choice' or ability to claim or express our personal power to change or escape our situations.

The adrenal dragon's solution to traumas of being overpowered is either to give up our power and learn to not notice, or not to care that we have no power, or to try to *overpower others before they overpower us.*

But our Spirit always feels and notices when we have no power, either consciously or subconsciously– even if we don't have the 'adrenal power' to do anything about it. And when we project this attitude in our energetic output by allowing others to *overpower us* or we when we *over power them* (the 'too much' and 'too little' of the adrenal energy), we are energetically in 'dragon territory.'

'Not noticing' or caring about having any personal power – or overpowering others, may be a great prison strategy (but prison guards are also prisoners in their environment). So remember the real question? How long do we want to 'live' or stay in the prison of *enduring our life without claiming or having any authentic personal power* (the kind that is 'just right') to show up and manifest our Spirit's path?

The emotional function of our adrenals is to instantly and clearly perceive power/pressure issues and be able to show up with courage to act in alignment with our Spirit's truth. When our adrenal function is healthy, we will not be reactively and unconsciously directed (in our present) by our past memories and feelings of shame from feeling we have no power to meet pressure with pressure to create feelings of pride – which can manifest as under-powering or over-powering. And if we 'miss the boat' on this, we will feel incapable of having authentic personal power in our life.

In other words, we are designed with the emotional ability to perceive and process the pressures of our life with feelings that are guided and directed by the Laws and Ways of energy. Love, compassion and courage guided by the Light of Truth gently lead us to that 'straight and narrow path' to our own authentic personal power.

'Drag' on our adrenal Spirit Life-force energy from memory of having no power dims our emotional feelings of being capable of expressing personal power because of how we mentally think and plan defensively by making decisions that are disempowering. This, in turn, feeds our adrenal drag, causing us to endure the shame of feeling disempowered and makes us incapable of meeting life's pressure with sufficient opposing pressure to be believable and effectively stand up for and defend our position. The key here is shame. The 'drag' on adrenal Spirit Life-force energy that we take on to endure the shame of having no power causes us to feel like giving up on our Spirit's desire for personal pride. Shame can take on many faces and it is what we end up with when we either under-power or overpower others.

The conscious, elegant solution that regenerates our adrenal energy is being consciously able to perceive and process the subtle aspects of our daily pressures clearly. We need to instantly know and effectively exert whatever pressure is necessary, in our moments of power, to feel our authentic power and express it so it gives our Spirit pride. We must be conscious enough to stay ahead of reactively reliving our dragon's unconscious shame from old dysfunctional patterns here and now from old memory of having no power.

These reactive un-cleared trauma memories that create adrenal issues often come from a history of enduring the shame of living without authentic power and feeling we are unable to change or escape from having no power or being overpowered.

Connecting with and following our adrenal Spirit Life-force energy to make decisions and take actions to claim our personal power (without being overpowering or being overpowered by triggered old feelings of shame) is regenerative. Such action gives us new memory for behavior that perpetuates feelings of personal pride within our Self. Anything less is not a sustainable adrenal strategy and will not lead to regenerative solutions.

14. Mind Spirit Function - Our Analyzer

Our mind Spirit Life-force energy gives us the ability to abstractly see and imagine conceptually how energetic Reality actually works, which gives us the ability to consciously see further ahead of the cure more clearly and quickly. This also allows us to figure out and understand certain energetic truths and how they come together in the moment to reveal and demonstrate the Ways of energetic Reality.

Being conscious clearly and quickly in this way and doing it consistently, requires that our concepts of understanding be an accurate reflection of energetic Reality that precisely aligns with the Laws and Ways of energetic Reality. With this view in our mind we can quickly figure out almost anything so long as we see it within the context of the Laws/Ways of energy, which will quickly reveal a clear picture of how things work so we know what to expect before we ever get there, with a fair degree of accuracy.

Our mind dragon dark-force energy comes from memories and imaginings of trauma experiences of needing to figure out survival plans, which have conditioned and programmed our unconscious reactive/survival memory to take over our mind functions with past defensive planning in our present life. However, defensive plans are only designed for survival to keep us ahead of what we fear while being directed by triggered and projected associated memory from our past.

This defensive plan instantly disconnects us from consciously being *'here now'* in full connection with present Reality and the Rules and Tools needed to run our life effectively – because defensive consciousness focuses us *'out there'* on what might happen *'then'* – when our own survival is at stake.

In our relationships, being present consistently is essential to being able to stay connected to what's happening in the *'here and now'* (where our best 'relating' takes place), through immediate experiences of what we perceive and express. We can't be fully present, here and now, when we are being unconsciously triggered by our present experiences to project our past memory into our future fears. This distracts us from any real connecting and is very detrimental to any real relationship.

Thinking and acting defensively causes one to feel cautious and especially careful about what one says or does, for fear of being criticized or made wrong by those who are around us. The result is internal conflict from mental worry focused on trying to plan ahead to make sure everything will be okay when we get there. All of this is done to try to predict and create a safe future at the cost of disconnecting from our present to try to ensure that we won't ever be 'made wrong' or be criticized by anyone ever again.

This whole defensive idea of not feeling safe and worthy of love just for being who we are, naturally creates pressure on our mind, because we feel we have to figure out everything before we get there and how it will turn out. If we don't, the dragon opportunistically tells us that it will be our fault because we didn't see or do something in advance before the 'wrong' thing happens. (And if we buy it we own it.)

This is our mind dragon's way of using our mind energy defensively to try to worry enough to create an immediate peace by trying to think of everything in advance. It does this by using up our mind's presence to analyze, calculate and figure out ahead of time so we can busily predict where and how and who is safe. This doesn't sound so bad, but it does this at the cost of being here now where our real personal power exists. And without being 'here now', we cannot be present enough to be capable of doing what really needs to be done now to win our life's energy game in the moment.

> *Remember the rule: If we need to be in defense,*
> *we shouldn't be there.*
> *If we don't need to be in defense,*
> *we shouldn't be in defense.*

Our mind works effectively for figuring out anything that can be understood by an *'if, then, therefore'* reasoning process of linear thinking (like math problems, the stock market, or for *abstract planning* to design a building). But if *inappropriately* used (for disconnected worry) this kind of thinking can be very self-destructive by distracting us from the *essential connecting needed* to maintain positive fulfilling personal relationships!

If you are always trying to figure out what's going to happen *there and then,* you can never be *here and now* (which is where real and meaningful human relationships always take place, right?). This is why very 'abstract people' with a high preference for being in their own abstract world often have problems in intimate relationships, because *nobody wants to have a relationship with anyone who isn't there.*

The mind's *defensive strategy* can only protect us 'in our present' *as we remember* it did 'in our past' by only using our mind's defensive memory to think ahead as a strategy for surviving and avoiding trauma.

The mind is about 'worry' or 'wonder.' The mind dragon's solution to traumas is to worry obsessively over unknowns, without using our mind's ability to wonder or imagine the many productive solutions to our problems before they occur in real time. The mind dragon may be totally consumed by focusing on how to avoid what we don't want by worrying about what's going to happen, rather than using our mind to wonder, imagine and proactively create solutions to what we do want.

Our mind's Spirit energy always notices, consciously or subconsciously what's really happening in our life – even if we don't have the mind power to do anything about how much we are consumed by our mind dragon's defensive focus on *worrying over unknowns* that create our own 'mental prison.'

Remember, the emotional function of our mind is to consciously and instantly feel the difference between our Spirit's mind function of creative curiosity or wonder – and the mind's dragon function of worry. It is designed with this ability to consciously feel this difference and use it to guide and direct us toward the creative wonder of creating solutions – and away from the degenerative worry of surviving unknown problems without solutions.

We must learn to find, stay and live where we feel safe. This involves following a plan that feels safe and worthy of love, without feeling we have to worry in order to survive!

Electrical 'drag' on our mind's Life-force energy (from worry over unknowns) dulls our emotional feelings and makes us less conscious of our mind's Spirit-ability to create regenerative solutions from focused, creative wonder about what our solutions could be. Besides, drag creates degenerative problems from focused worry over unknowns we can't do anything about – except to make ourselves worse.

In summary, our mind energy can be used either for creative *wonder,* to create productive, fulfilling regenerative sustainable solutions for our future, or for *worry,* to figure out how to defensively survive our problems. This defensive position leaves us without the ability to create solutions, while living where we don't feel safe or worthy of love.

The 'drag' that we take on from *worry* to endure and survive what we *fear* can consume almost all of our mental energy with none left to inspire the *wonder* of our imagination from our Spirit Life-force energy that will (when used properly) create our elegant solutions that eliminate our problems.

The conscious, elegant solution for our Spirit's mind energy comes from being able to clearly, quickly and appropriately focus our creative ability to wonder, perceive and direct regenerative decisions and actions that create elegant solutions for our future – without creating degenerative problems from worry over unknowns and hopeless problems we have no way of solving.

The un-cleared trauma memory that creates mind dragon issues comes from a history of feeling we have to endure and survive unknowns that we can't figure out. This defensive plan helps us to continue to endure not feeling safe and worthy of love while living in fear and worry over future unknowns without being able to imagine what is needed for us to escape our situation.

When we are in a habit of worrying compulsively over unknowns, this defensive behavior consumes our mind's Life-force energy for what often turns out to be bogus survival issues at the expense of our Spirit's wonder – *which is the real secret to imagining and creating our fulfilling elegant solutions!*

Connecting with our mind's ability to *wonder and imagine solutions* allows us to see and make decisions that cause us to feel safe enough in the moment to actually 'be here now' so we can create solutions that work energetically. Our mind's sustainable and regenerative solution strategy is to use our *imagination* to first figure out our solutions and then focus on connecting the dots that give them form to become real.

15. Hypothalamus Spirit Function - Our Attender

Our hypothalamus Spirit Life-force energy gives us the ability to clearly *attend* to what we sense from what we *see, hear, taste, touch and smell.* Attending is more than just seeing and perceiving something, it is about giving it attention. As we become better able to attend, we become more conscious of the refined subtle aspects of our five senses, and we also develop a greater 'sixth sense.' This *extra sensory perception* gives us the ability to attend to the more subtle intuitive energies *beyond the visible spectrum* of the 'rainbow' (the rainbow only contains the denser third-dimensional physical world).

Tuning in to the subtle aspects of energetic Reality provides us with what we call our 'intuition' – our *ability to accurately 'read between the lines'* of our senses to see how the bigger picture of energetic Reality connects with the more subtle aspects of what's really happening. This is how we 'see things' and 'put things together' that we can't explain from third-dimensional concepts and observations.

But in the end, when the bigger subtle-energy picture is revealed through all of our senses being 'in synch' at once, it all 'comes together' and energetic Reality always clearly 'makes sense' because there is no other possibility since *everything is energy and energy always follows the Laws and Ways of energy.*

Clarity is a powerful tool, because when we become conscious of the full spectrum of sensory and extra-sensory energy, this view clarifies major confusions and distortions of Reality. These are the same distortions that often confuse much of our daily communication so our thoughts are completely disconnected from actual energetic Reality.

We need precise refined abstract conceptual pictures in our mind founded on clear accurate perceptions of energetic Reality in order to clearly see, understand and communicate energetic Reality clearly to others. (A requirement to begin any successful accomplishment is that we must accept Reality and follow it.) This requires sufficient hypothalamus consciousness (without drag) to be able to tune in to and perceive our 'here and now' Reality with our sixth sense to see our clearest most complete perceptions.

Without drag, our hypothalamus Spirit Life-force energy gives us the ability to focus our attention on what we need to 'see' to *create the results we desire*. This also requires refined conscious *perceptions* of our sensory input to clearly define energetic Reality.

When such clear perceptions of our sensory inputs occur and are acted upon, they produce results because the perceptions that are guiding us are aligned with energetic Reality and thus direct our actions to flow in alignment with producing the results we desire.

But the hypothalamus energy is not just about attending to what our senses are feeding us. It is about the process of communicating as well. We must *conceptualize* and articulate accurate *perceptions* of Reality into our *language* so we can *communicate* clear perceptions of what is real.

If we have clear conceptual perceptions that are effectively articulated, we can better understand and *communicate* our subtle-energy realms of consciousness. This is the only chance we have to create the *results* that are possible when we perceive and align with energetic Reality – which is our Spirit's desire.

The *hypothalamus dragon* enters the picture when our hypothalamus Life-force energy is programmed and conditioned with drag from trauma memories of feeling we must *inhibit our communication and distort our perceptions* of Reality to learn to see 'reality' *'as it is not'* to adapt to an environment not harmonious with our Spirit. This creates a *'bubble reality' (little 'r' – which is not the complete picture)*.

The *hypothalamus dragon's mastery* is designed to unconsciously *distort* our perceptions of energetic Reality by projecting past memory of past reality as 'experienced *then*' onto what's actually happening *now* in energetic Reality. Consciousness is always about *getting ahead of the dragon's* triggered unconscious curves (in this case it is about the limited, self centered ideas about Reality that define the 'dragon's bubble').

This life is a game where we learn about what is real and what is unreal, energetically. A clear perception of energetic Reality *always reveals the more subtle and refined aspects of our problems and solutions* because the Laws of energy don't work according to our beliefs. They work according to the laws of energy. Conscious alignment with ener-getic Reality is essential in order to effectively function in a world where we all must live. Staying out of the bubbles of distortion and staying in our present makes all the difference energetically, no matter what we think we know or believe.

Not noticing the refined aspects of our problems and solutions from inadequate, distracted and distorted attending, comes from hypo-thalamus drag, from trauma memory of being, feeling and/or think-ing in inhibited ways, which causes our learning to spin backward defensively.

At this point, our defensive philosophy becomes: "Since I must be inhibited in order to feel safe, how is the best way to live my life?" The dragon does this to protect us from communicating authentically in an unsafe inauthentic environment by distorting our reality to match what we are supposed to see or be – to avoid exposing it like it is and being real.

When our dragons rule by *a strategy of distorting Reality* as our default position, we end up living as 'ideas of ourselves' rather than as our authentic selves. We are surrounded in the bubble of an 'idea' (a hypothetical construct) of what we call 'reality' or what the group we are in calls 'reality'. Like attracts like as we find ourselves with other people who agree with our construct – rather than consciously living in *actual energetic Reality as it naturally exists.* When we follow this energetically backward perspective, we can easily come to believe, reinforce, enable and maintain our own distortions of energetic Reality. What we feel and think seems to matter less and less as we try to align with the 'tribe' rather than our own feelings and instincts.

When we continue to believe in our distortions, we become invested in our distortions and their interests. We then have to distort Reality (see things the way they *'are not'* and *'not hear'* things the way *'they are,'* etc.) to *defend our distortions.* The hypothalamus dragon's magic power comes from making us *unconscious* of 'what is real' and *conscious* of 'what is not real' without being able to tell the difference between energetic Reality and seeing and living our distortions!

The hypothalamus dragon's solution is to survive environments that inhibit our Spirit from perceiving and communicating our truth, by dis-associating us from our energetic sensory Reality to protect us from 'sensory' abuse. It does this by creating a drag on our conscious awareness of our hypothalamus Spirit Life-force that clearly perceives Reality as it is.

This is the organ that processes our sensory input. This is why this particular dragon distorts the clarity of not only our sensory but our extra-sensory perceptions of Reality in order to allow us to distort and ignore Reality. It might even feel it necessary to make-up a new 'reality' (and that's when the distortion becomes the 'new reality.' At this point, the dragon will assist us to see what perception of reality is *needed* to fit the situation or to *not see* what isn't convenient (in order to feel safe).

This is how well meaning people end up lying or fooling themselves and staying in denial of Realities that may be obvious to everyone around them but leave them 'clueless' to the inconvenient truths!

It's how they even end up believing their own distortions (especially if they have gone through a great deal of trouble in making them up to 'fit' the situation)! Just remember, the dragon will always try to sell you anything you will 'buy.' The problem ends up being about feeling and believing *we must endure and survive* what is not real because we believe we cannot change or escape it.

Our Spirit always notices when our clear perceptions are being ignored (either consciously or subconsciously – even if it doesn't have the 'hypothalamus power' to do anything about it). When our hypothalamus is flowing with Spirit Life-force energy, it discriminates and feels the prison walls of distorted thinking from twisted perceptions. It sees through whatever is blocking real, authentic connections through communication.

If our hypothalamus Spirit Life-force energy is unconsciously directed by triggered trauma (dragon) memory of inhibited perceptions and communications, our senses are distorted with projected negative sensory memory to defensively prepare for present experiences to be like our past associated memory.

Consequently, if the dragon controls our decisions and actions we will act in the *present* as if we are reliving our *past* by projecting that memory to make our decisions in our *present*.

Our (conscious or unconscious) *protection reactions* are triggered when our dragon notices any 'red flags' of *old familiar feelings* of being unsafe when we are *real*. These come from present triggers of old *associations* with past trauma memory when we were not safe being real. The real question is whether the *present* experience is the *same or different* from the past associated triggered memories?

We can usually only determine what the true answer is by sufficient effective free and open communication that is refined and sensitive enough to reveal the truth. This can only really be accomplished by consciously staying out of reaction energetically while effectively *communicating* our truth while clearly *observing* their Spirit's response and dragon reactions to our truth.

Otherwise, the hypothalamus dragons (our own and those of others), disconnect us from 'here and now' sensory Reality by distorting and inhibiting real 'here and now' perceptual connections with Reality. This disables our ability to focus our attention on anything that feels 'too real,' or ever to be able to focus on creating what we really want and need to get the results our Spirit desires.

When we attend to our triggered sensory trauma memory, we create an 'attention deficit.' This is because our attention is disconnected because we don't feel safe paying attention to what's happening 'here now' because it was not safe then, so it does not feel safe to show up real now. When this happens, the feeling is: "Why bother?"

This is our hypothalamus dragon's defensive thinking strategy of disconnecting from negative energy in order to protect us from sensory trauma in the present based on our past. An example of this is what happens when a child is repeatedly screamed at over a long period of time. After awhile the child learns to 'tune it out' rather than actually 'tune in' to what feels bad about what the person is saying.

This is our hypothalamus defense against being overwhelmed by excess sensory stimulation from unpleasant physical and/or emotional sensory energy being radiated on us. This is how sensory overload is created on all of our senses. Some other examples of sensory radiation are hearing anything that is too loud, a baby crying incessantly, feeling 'bad vibes' from a person, seeing things that are upsetting to you, smelling things that are nauseating, tasting things that are offensive, etc.

The defensive maneuver of shutting down our sensory input and disconnecting ourselves from our 'here and now' when necessary is defensively functional. But it also creates a drag on our essential ability to open up and pay attention to and focus on our sensory input that is required to be able to discern the finer and finer differences that give us clearer Real perceptions in order to create the results we desire.

The drag on our hypothalamus Spirit Life-force energy causes us to lose hope for our Spirit desire to feel safe perceiving Reality clearly and communicating about it freely. Instead, we end up treating the situation as if it were 'ok' to not feel safe expressing our true feelings.

Our Spirit's conscious elegant solution for using our hypothalamus energy is to feel and be safe and able to consciously perceive energetic Reality. Then, we can use that clarity to direct our life to align with the subtle Ways of energy that produce regenerative outcomes from following clear perceptions and communications. And we can more effectively do this without degenerative, inhibited and distorted perceptions of reality that cause disruptive miscommunications.

The emotional function of the hypothalamus attends to and perceives the feeling differences between inhibited communication (feeling shut down and disconnected), versus being able to feel safe, clear, free and real in the 'here and now.' These feeling differences dramatically and directly affect whether or not we can communicate freely and connect openly to portray our true perceptions of Reality.

185

We are emotionally designed to use these feeling differences to determine how we communicate with others. This is how we are consciously guided to direct our in the moment communications with others. One thing to note here is that not everyone *feels safe* to talk to because some are *not safe* to talk to. These observational skills can also assist us in discerning who we can talk openly with and who is not safe to talk openly with. Also, we can more clearly discern 'why or why not' we feel the ways we do in our personal interactions.

'Drag' on our hypothalamus Life-force energy diminishes our ability to emotionally connect with our truth and discern distortions of energetic Reality clearer and quicker to stay consciously connected with clear perceptions that accurately reflect energetic Reality through our communications.

Our hypothalamus's energy either fulfills our desires with clear uninhibited communications – or we defensively survive and endure unclear, distorted perceptions and communications as our way of life.

The bottom line is that if one cannot hold a clear focus on Reality, then one cannot efficiently and effectively create and produce regenerative results in their lives. This organ's energy is all about our focus of attention – and as a result it is largely responsible for what we are able to effectively create or not.

(This issue of attention and focus is sometimes confused with the liver issue which is about creating what we want from the focus of attention. So, here is a test for your hypothalamus – to attend to and focus on the finer differences while they are being explained (so you can communicate about them later)! The liver issue is about a sustainability of focus to transmute or create what you want and the hypothalamus is about the clarity of focus needed to communicate it so you can create what you want.)

The un-cleared trauma memories that create hypothalamus issues come from a history of traumas to our senses (like somebody beating us or yelling at us). They could also come from more subtle emotional assaults that cause us not to trust believing in and feeling good about expressing our real perceptions of Reality. This, in turn, causes us to feel inhibited in how we perceive and communicate with our outside world, which dramatically affects our ability to ever feel safe enough to get clear enough to be able to direct our life so we do the actions necessary to create the results our Spirit desires.

Connecting with and following our hypothalamus Spirit's truth allows us to choose those persons who make our Spirit feel safe enough to allow us to perceive and communicate clearly enough to consciously get ahead of our distorted perceptions of Reality. This is the only sustainable and regenerative strategy that will inevitably solve hypothalamus problems of defensively living with distorted and inhibited perceptions of Reality.

16. Kidneys and Bladder Spirit Function - Our Purifier

Our kidney Spirit Life-force energy gives us the ability to *filter refuse from our body's fluids and our life's experiences* to purify and clarify our finer discriminations of feelings for what is 'pure' and what 'needs to be refused' or filtered from our life.

Our kidney Spirit Life-force energy perceptions and expressions of filtering are designed to remove what is not pure or right for us emotionally because it goes against our Spirit's Ways.

Filtering requires consciously getting ahead of our triggered reactive drag from projecting old unconscious memories into our decisions in our moments of power. This degenerative habit is a result of enduring the toxic emotional situations from unconscious trauma memory.

To filter, we must first be able to consciously *perceive* what doesn't work for us emotionally and then be able to *express* (filter and/or say) what doesn't work for us emotionally. Expressing this filtering effectively in a timely manner is the key, because *only our performance counts* for results. Performance means appropriately expressing clearly, quickly and appropriately to effectively and efficiently filter out what is *not* pure from what *is* pure in our life.

The Spirit Life-force energy of the kidney system gives us the ability to purify ourselves. It does this by filtering out or *refusing* what is not pure – confronting the impurities we encounter to prevent them from creating a drag on our Spirit's ability to follow what feels right emotionally.

We need to *feel safe* to follow our Spirit's purity to be authentic and regenerative in our emotional interactions with each other.

Fear is the emotional issue of the kidney and bladder energy. You might ask how fear works as a filter. The answer is that the feeling of *fear* allows us to *feel what works for us emotionally and what doesn't.* If we feel our kidney Spirit function, we can tune in very quickly to what doesn't work for us emotionally.

So, in other words – when it is used as designed, fear is actually needed to purify our life and body from toxic fluids and emotional situations because *fear tells us to filter.* If, however we have been traumatized and hold old memories of when we *felt we had to endure toxic emotional situations,* this *numbs* our fear or *makes us consumed by fear* and either way this makes us dysfunctional in terms of filtering effectively. This type of trauma memory aligns with a 'drag' on kidney functions.

So, fear is the key to the Spirit function of the kidney depending on how we use it. If our kidney Spirit function is traumatized, we tend to *overuse it or underuse it.* We underuse it by ignoring it and we overuse it by fearing anything and everything. Confronting toxic emotional situations with the appropriate filtering by expressing what 'does not work for us emotionally' purifies these emotional situations (or makes clear to us who really cares about what works for us emotionally).

But if, because of fear, we cannot confront toxic emotional situations with discernment and expression that purifies our situations, we will remain poisoned by this toxic energy.

The kidney dragon enters the picture when our kidney Life-force energy is programmed and conditioned to endure the drag of traumas and memories of having to ignore certain toxic emotional situations.

The kidney dragon inhibits our ability to discern the differences between what feels pure and safe to our Spirit and what does not. Not noticing these differences because of drag on the kidneys, programs us to defensively endure and survive without filtering toxic emotional situations out of our life.

The kidney dragon solution to toxic emotional situations is to *procrastinate* dealing with these situations by avoiding them and not noticing them, rather than immediately confronting them and filtering out *what is not pure from what is pure* in order to keep our life aligned with what works emotionally for us.

Our Spirit *always* notices when we don't purify our toxic emotional situations either consciously or subconsciously – even if it doesn't have the 'kidney power' to do anything about it.

When Spirit Life-force is flowing through the kidney, our Spirit keenly feels the 'toxic walls' of our own prison being created by enduring *impure situations* that enclose us in suppressed *feelings from fears* of confronting and filtering them out of our life.

But if we are able to *move past our fear* and simply express what does and does not work for us, we will have the power to filter those situations from our lives.

Kidney/bladder Spirit Life-force energy can be unconsciously programmed and directed by the dragon's projected reactive memory to not feel safe or able to confront our fears of filtering. This leaves us without the ability to filter out the many situations in our lives that are emotionally poisonous to us.

***Not filtering causes us to hold onto our toxic situation**s* and endure poisonous energy without purification, which spins our kidney energy backward, making us less able to notice and filter out toxic emotional situations. This continuously adds to our emotional debt with negative energy that numbs our feelings so we are more able to endure even more poisons and toxic emotional situations.

This, in turn, increases our tolerance for enduring toxic emotional situations without confronting or filtering what really needs to be purified. This creates a drag on kidney Spirit Life-force energy flow that results in increased toxicity in our emotional life and body fluids.

The emotional function of the kidney is designed to allow us to perceive the appropriate feelings of fear without experiencing too much and/or not enough fear to properly deal with emotional situations in our present Reality.

In other words, we are designed with the ability to feel the appropriate amount of fear and be consciously directed in our performances by clear and refined discernments for what is worthy of fear.

Drag on the kidney Life-force energy diminishes and distorts our emotional decrement for what is 'appropriate to fear' and what is 'not appropriate to fear.' The kidney function is designed to serve as a Reality-based filter that quickly knows the right amount of fear for what does/doesn't need to be feared. This Reality-based filter all depends on our circuits being connected – so they are free to receive Spirit Life-force input.

Inappropriate fears lead to procrastination. They disable our ability to effectively filter out toxic physical and emotional situations from our life, because we either experience too much or not enough fear to appropriately deal with certain emotional situations in a timely manner, without procrastinating blindly until we get into real trouble.

When we take on drag on the kidney Life-force energy, it diminishes our desire and ability to effectively filter toxic emotional situations out of our life. We no longer feel the urge to clearly and effectively communicate our true feelings so we can see who really cares about our true feelings or not. And sadly, without this ability, we don't have any idea who and what to filter out.

Our *kidney's* conscious elegant emotional solution is first being able to consciously perceive what doesn't work for us emotionally and then to be able to effectively express our truth clearly, quickly and appropriately in order to find and filter out what needs to be refused.

The un-cleared trauma memory that creates kidney issues comes from a history of feeling we must *endure toxic emotional situations* rather that express our emotional truth. This enables, creates and maintains our fears of confronting and 'filtering' toxic emotional situations from our life. We may see 'not filtering' as our only choice, because we have never been able to confront, change or escape past toxic emotional situations, and whenever we have tried to do so, it always seemed to just make them worse.

Connecting with and expressing our kidney Spirit's truth about what works for us and what does not work for us consistently filters and minimizes having to continually endure and survive toxic emotional situations. In filtering, expressing and following our true feelings we filter out energy that, if not filtered out, is unsustainable and degenerative and may inevitably lead to kidney problems.

17/18. Endocrine System Spirit Function - Our Balancer

Remember, the two numbers (17 and 18) represent this unique system because the endocrine system functions on two different levels. These two different levels of Spirit Life-force energy must always maintain an integrated balance: the *invisible* subtle-energy chakras, and the *visible* dense-energy endocrine glands. These emphasize energetically how our endocrine system performs our most critical function (which is to maintain homeostasis). The endocrine system does this by balancing critical glands, hormones, and chakras to energetically keep our

190

Spirit's Life-force energy connected to our physical body so we can stay alive.

These specific endocrine glands are designed to quickly *achieve and maintain continuous homeostasis* to keep our Spirit's Life-force energy connected to our physical body, which is what keeps us alive. Our endocrine Spirit Life-force energy maintains our physical-etheric homeostasis, moment-to-moment, between our subtle energy chakra levels and our dense physical gland level of energy functions.

These two distinct levels of energy are specifically designed to maintain an integrated homeostasis for the entire system by balancing our seven chakras [see chakras' image] of Life-force energies that flow in, out and through our twenty-three organ/gland energy systems to keep all of them in balance.

These seven endocrine glands (7-pineal, 6-pituitary, 5-thyroid, 4-thymus, 3-pancreas, 2-sex organs, 1-adrenals) integrate with our entire system. They are listed from the least refined (1) to the most refined energy (7). Scientifically, there is much yet to learn about the pineal gland, but what we do know so far is how astounding it is in many different aspects in regards to consciousness. Something also worth mentioning again here is that the pineal gland is specifically known for having refined *light sensitivity.*

The endocrine system's Spirit Life-force energy gives us the ability to recover and maintain 'energy balance' (homeostasis) in the face of unbalancing forces of trauma that destabilize our critical electromagnetic balance (homeostasis) – *needed every moment* to keep us alive.

In order to survive the endocrine system Spirit function will spontaneously take over our body when necessary to attend to our survival needs on all different energy levels and maintain homeostasis in the process with its seven levels of energy glands.

Doing this appropriately requires us to stay *consciously* ahead of the endocrine dragon to avoid *unconsciously* following triggered old habits that cause us to unnecessarily continue 'living in' and 'acting out' past trauma memory, which the endocrine dragon loves to do!

We need to keep ahead of this consciously to avoid unconsciously and reactively going down that familiar, endless degenerative path of surviving and enduring by just living in trauma.

Operating continuously from unconsciously triggered trauma memory out of our lower chakras provides short term plans for survival – which if hectic enough will override consciously being Who

We Are from our higher chakra' Spirit plans that provide long-term fulfillment plans.

Spirit plans seek to maintain sustainable regenerative balance from foresight to avoid engaging in unnecessary trauma that can be avoided. What it takes is being more conscious of this art of balancing for survival while evolving to consciously be further ahead of the curve quicker, clearer and more often.

But first, this requires us to be sufficiently conscious to be able to tune in to the higher resonance of our more subtle aspects of energetic Reality quickly – and then to take the appropriate action to enact our most effective long-term solutions from being directed by our clarity for energetic Reality.

Our endocrine system energy must regain balance from the unbalancing effects of traumas, in order for us to stay alive every moment. If our homeostatic balance is *not* almost immediately restored, our Spirit's Life-force energy breaks connection with our physical body's organs and glands. And without our Spirit's Life-force energy connected to our body, we physically *die!*

Our endocrine Spirit Life-force energy can be conditioned, programmed and directed by triggered unconscious 'dragon memory' of feeling we need to *'walk on eggshells'* – which amounts to continuously *living in trauma.*

This can become such a habit that is so familiar, we unconsciously *live in this memory of trauma,* where everything is always an emergency that requires an immediate short-term solution (which itself creates *degeneration* and more long-term problems from exhaustion and depletion that come from living without a long-term plan that creates and maintains *regeneration*).

Triggered *'relives'* of our time-warped memories of living in trauma cause us to feel like we are in a continuous state of panic about our survival, which further triggers other associated memories of similar traumas. Such continuous experiences create physical and emotional hormonal imbalances in our body.

The endocrine system dragon enters the picture when our endocrine Life-force energy system is programmed and conditioned by memory of having to live in trauma (this plays out later as the feeling that we must endure living in trauma). These experiences trigger, enable and maintain even more trauma memory that creates even more drag on our endocrine system energy.

Over time, this drag dulls our perceptions for quickly discerning the feeling differences between (1) Regenerative homeostasis, and (2) Degenerative homeostasis so we may learn better to avoid the latter. These general differences are described below:

(1) Regenerative homeostasis has to do with staying out of war zones and staying Spirit centered and safe by avoiding engagement with dragons.

Our long-term regenerative homeostasis begins by learning to avoid war zones, where the best we can do is survive without hope for fulfillment, while we degenerate moment-by-moment. We must learn to avoid the war torn areas of our lives if Spirit has communicated to us that there is nothing we can do about them so we can feel safe to become centered within.

Focusing on externals to try to feel safe isn't the same as an internal Spirit centered and driven focus. But we cannot get to this point without feeling safe. *When we feel safe and worthy of love,* we can begin to connect with our Self to find and follow our path toward regenerative homeostasis.

If and when we engage with negative/dragon forces we automatically become part of the problem because ***engagement with negative forces reinforces, enables and maintains the dragon's ways of survival***.

(2) Degenerative homeostasis is about short term safety at the expense of our long term regeneration.

Our short-term degenerative homeostasis is for when we ***must be where it is unsafe*** like war zones where the focus is on armor, bullets and defensive expertise to counterbalance whatever diabolical traumatic perversions may oppose us.

This is all done at the expense of our total Life-force energy (because defense is degenerative and non-productive), but it must be respected because it enables us to survive our war zone moments (or our entire lives if we live in war zones and haven't yet figured out how to get out of them).

Knowing the differences between regenerative and degenerative homeostasis makes us more capable of avoiding degeneration. In order to avoid degeneration we must consciously function ahead of the endocrine gland dragon curve. This means first becoming consciously aware of how we engage in unnecessary trauma just because it's familiar. Secondly – by knowing our truth.

This allows us to know when and how to express what to whom in order to make things work effectively and productively. Otherwise, if we operate without clear centered direction we will unconsciously spin our energy backward defensively (out of confusion and fear) to protect ourselves even if we don't need it.

The endocrine system dragon solution is to disconnect from our Spirit by becoming hyper-involved in the 'trauma' so nothing else can enter our consciousness. But our Spirit always notices when its truth is being ignored either consciously or subconsciously – even if it doesn't have the 'endocrine power' to do anything about it.

And when Spirit Life-force is flowing through our endocrine system, it will usually tell us where we shouldn't go when we are listening. And we will instantly be acutely aware that it is not regenerative to enter the endocrine dragon prison of making decisions that result in continuously living in trauma.

Remember: at times there are legitimate 'traumas' that enter our lives that are indeed life threatening.

The emotional function of the endocrine system is to perceive, feel and be guided and directed by the differences between traumas that are critically necessary to deal with immediately, versus traumas that are not worth engaging with because they will enable and maintain the dragons.

'Drag' on endocrine system Life-force energy lessens our ability to discriminate between acute essential traumas that we must deal with, and chronic distorted traumas that we unconsciously create and maintain from reliving triggered dragon memories and engaging in non productive emotional trauma drama.

Defensively using our endocrine energy to survive living in trauma consumes vast amounts of Life-force. If we have a conscious choice to not engage in and endure such continuing traumas in our life, and yet we still do – we must ask ourselves – who is really running our life?

In summary, the conscious, elegant solution for our endocrine system energy is to consciously perceive and direct us to avoid traumas unless absolutely necessary (instead of playing into trauma, which then justifies and maintains trauma).

The un-cleared trauma memory that creates endocrine system issues comes from a history of enduring and surviving traumas where we feel we have no other choice.

Connecting with and following our endocrine system Spirit energy allows us to see clearer and stay further ahead of the dragon's curves quicker so we can maintain long-term regenerative balance and avoid having to engage in, survive and/or endure unnecessary traumas.

The elegant solution, of course, is consciousness which allows us to avoid unnecessary traumas by choosing not to participate in them. Doing this is the most basic regenerative strategy for preventing physical hormone/endocrine problems and the emotional effects of living in 'trauma memory prison.'

19. Skin Spirit Function - Our Identifier

Our skin Spirit Life-force energy gives us the ability to feel safe and secure *defining, defending and expressing our true identity.* Our skin Life-force energy also establishes our physical and emotional boundaries with the outside world. This energy allows us to feel safe and worthy of love just being who we are, so we can feel secure defining, defending and expressing our true identity.

When we feel safe and comfortable *being in our skin,* then we may begin to learn to consciously function being true to our Self by operating ahead of our triggered curves of reactive decisions and actions of codependence that overshadow our true identity. Sometimes we lose ourselves to the point where we are driven by what others want, at the expense of what our true Self wants, which is how we lose our identity.

Codependence is avoided when we learn to feel safe consciously following our skin Spirit Life-force energy's desire to express our true Self's identity. Expressing our true Self requires sufficient consciousness to first tune in to Who we are as our true 'Spirit Self' identity, with our unique talents and special God-given gifts. These individual talents and gifts define our true identity and challenge us to fulfill our divine intent that no other person has in the exact same way.

As we become conscious of the drag on expressing our true identity (clearly, quickly and appropriately), we learn to connect to our truth from our inside world and then connect our truth to the outside world.

When we learn to perform in accordance with our true identity, effectively, it shows in our body language. Our body language shows our personal power when we are coming from a loving intent, with a quest for the truth and a great sense of humor while not taking things too personally or too seriously.

Who we are also shows up in our smile when it is connected to our truth (in what I call a 'Mona Lisa' smile of contented connection with our true Self). On the other hand, a 'dragon smile' is a smile of deception used to hide our truth, our Self, and our feelings.

[Author's note: Personal papers of Leonardo Da Vinci, the painter of the Mona Lisa, called her "La Gioconda," which is Italian for "jocund," "happy" or "jovial." Art historians throughout the decades have seen Mona Lisa's smile as being mysterious, enigmatic and ambiguous. I see it as being a contented smile of being at peace with her truth, her Self, and her true feelings which is why I use 'the Mona Lisa smile' in this way. Also, for a long time, nobody knew her identity – but in 2005 it was confirmed who she was (https://en.wikipedia.org/wiki/Mona_ Lisa). So, it is even more appropriate to refer to this 'lost' woman as we discuss our Spirit identities and how we can so easily 'lose them' as well as find our desire to fulfill our divine intent by expressing our talents and unique innate abilities, like how 'Leonardo' did!]

Our skin Spirit Life-force energy is designed to enable us to claim our true identity and defend it by demarcating personal boundaries that define and express the character of our 'true Self identity.' Our skin energy defines who we are in terms of what we present to the outside world, and how we perform, portray, define, defend and express our true identity. This is all determined by how we express and perform in the 'movie of our life' to make our own unique contribution (divine intent) to our world.

If not, our 'drag' on skin Spirit Life-force energy programs and directs our identity with drag from the old unconscious trauma memory of feeling unsafe being our true Self identity. When this happens, this energy can take over our true identity by programming us to disassociate from our true Self and either lose our identity – or identify with someone else's identity. We do this as an attempt to feel safe by trying to become what they think we should be. But this defensive 'safety' cannot provide long term success.

If we repeat this pattern of trying to become what others think we should be, we will *feel even more and more unsafe owning and expressing our own true identity,* which results in continuing to have feelings of *lost identity.* This experience of never feeling safe to know, be and express who we really are can easily result in becoming codependent. We can do this to the point that we never feel safe enough to define, defend and express our true identity.

When skin identity energy is traumatized and defensively programmed, we deny and tend to give up our identity in order to support someone else's identity (which further contributes to our own sense of lost identity). In other words, it seems easier and safer to identify with someone else's identity and endure the boredom of doing 'somebody else's thing' instead of doing 'our own thing.' The dragon mind-set is: "What's important to someone else – is more important to us." This versus what is really important to us!

The skin dragon enters the picture when our skin Life-force energy becomes conditioned and programmed by the 'drag' on our skin from trauma memory of lost identity and living someone else's identity. This comes from not feeling safe to define, defend and express our own true Self. This reinforces enables and maintains codependency, which further weakens our ability to stand up for Who we really are as Spirit and express our differences between someone else's identity and our own true identity.

Not noticing or expressing our true identity causes us to spin our identity energy backward to defensively better endure and survive feeling lost by doing now what we had to do then. The skin dragon's solution to 'identity challenges' is to not notice our lost identity, but instead to just follow another's identity, helping them to be who they are or get what they want.

Our Spirit always notices when it is being ignored, either consciously or subconsciously– even if it doesn't have the 'skin power' to do anything about it. But when Spirit Life-force is flowing through our skin circuits, we know exactly Who we are. Ignoring our Spirit's true identity creates a 'skin dragon prison' of living someone else's life at the expense of our own identity.

The emotional function of our skin energy gives us the ability to perceive the feeling differences between living according to our true identity and living other people's identity. In other words, we have the emotional ability to feel like we are *winning* when we are connected with our true self and feeling safe to define, defend and express 'Who' we really are. And when we don't do this, we feel like we are *losing* (because we are losing our identity).

'Drag' on our skin Life-force energy weakens our emotional discrimination for *tuning into* doing our own thing versus doing someone else's thing, which eventually will lead to boredom – a signal that is telling us we are *not doing our own thing.*

The 'drag' on our Spirit Life-force skin energy that we take on in order to survive not feeling safe to be Who we are causes us to lose our desire and ability to maintain a healthy personal identity. The conscious, elegant, emotional solution for our skin Life-force energy is to be able to stay consciously connected to and directed by our true Self (without playing unconscious dragon games of being directed by another's identity, at the expense of our own identity).

The un-cleared trauma memory that creates skin issues comes from a history of *having to endure lost identity in an environment where our identity was and is not valued, supported or nourished.* Disconnecting from knowing and following our skin Spirit's Life-force that maintains our boundaries and defines our true identity – forces us to survive by living someone else's view of our identity. This is an unsustainable and degenerative strategy that will manifest as skin and identity issues and problems in our life and body!

20. Pancreas Spirit Function - Our Expressionist

Our pancreas Spirit Life-force energy function gives us the ability to consciously connect with, perceive and express our own true feelings, which are designed to guide and direct us to perform our divine intent by both knowing and following our true feelings that give us joy and laughter.

Our true feelings, when appropriately perceived, expressed and followed, guide and direct us to all of our divine intentions. Doing what aligns with our truth invokes in us the feeling of joy that comes from locating and following our divine intent – which is what gives us true inspiration (being 'in Spirit').

The pancreas Spirit Life-force energy gives us the ability to consciously feel and express our own true feelings. This requires being able, in the moment, to consciously get ahead of old triggered familiar unconscious reactive habits that quietly suppress and hide our true feelings with various cover-ups.

We learn to follow our true feelings by first consciously accepting them!

Then, effective expression of our true feelings requires us to perform in accordance with how we feel, so that our feelings align with what we 'say and do,' clearly and quickly. Then it is all about how appropriately we perform in our life to be effective and productive in our outcome.

The pancreas dragon enters the picture when our pancreas Life-force energy gets programmed and conditioned with drag from memory of not feeling safe expressing our true feelings, which unconsciously suppresses our true feelings from being expressed and followed in order to manifest our divine intent.

The pancreas dragon weakens our conscious perceptions for knowing the difference between our true feelings and those we make up to pretend we feel. There is a cause and effect to everything. Not noticing these real differences between our true and untrue feelings is the effect of 'drag' that is set off by triggered past trauma memory of not feeling safe expressing and following our true feelings.

These defensively triggered suppressive actions spin our pancreas energy backward to endure and survive by suppressing our true feelings. The pancreas dragon's solution is suppressing our true feelings by not noticing what our true feelings really are so we never remember to express them when we need to.

But our Spirit always notices when its pancreas truth is being ignored either consciously or subconsciously– even if it doesn't have the pancreas power to do anything about it. But when Spirit Life-force pancreas energy is flowing freely without drag so we feel safe expressing our true feelings, we have no problem processing everything in our life clearly, quickly and appropriately. This is how we stay connected to our Self through our true feelings.

Ignoring our pancreas Spirit's Life-force (our true feelings) creates our pancreas dragon's prison walls by dislocating and walling us off from *suppressed feelings that dissociate us*. When this occurs, we *cannot consciously connect* with and follow our true feelings that guide and direct us to our divine intent.

Following our pancreas feelings eventually leads us to the *sweetness in our life* – which is our *divine intent* that comes from our true Spirit connection! Great love connections involve laughter and joy. This Spirit connection in the long run is what makes real relationships a worthy endeavor.

What I have noticed is that when two people are 'getting real' – even if there are strong emotions involved – that the 'realness' is what brings them to a reciprocal 'love response' which leads to laughter and joy. But it cannot happen between two people if only one person is committed to being real.

Our suppressed expression and dissociations (which are also dislocations from our true feelings) causes a hunger for the sweetness of life. One of our dragon's short-term degenerative solutions is to substitute the feeling of sweetness from sugar, which can develop into sugar cravings.

These suppressed expressions of our emotions result in physical cravings that drive us to eat sweets for temporary fixes to sweeten our life. This is to counterbalance feeling disconnected from our true Self and the people that we need to express our true feelings to.

This disconnection is our defensive strategy that causes us to not follow our true feelings. This leaves us with the end result of a depression (from the root word 'pressure'). This deep pressure has usually been building for quite some time before it emerges into chronic depression.

This result is losing our desire and ability to stay connected to, and true to, our feelings. As this continues, we become even more disconnected and depressed from our lack of real sweetness in our life.

In summation, our pancreas emotional function is our ability to perceive, discern and express our true feelings quickly, which is essential for us to be able to *consciously guide and direct our true Self* according to our authentic feelings.

The conscious, elegant, emotional solution for our pancreas Lifeforce energy is being able to consciously perceive and direct our path by *following our true feelings,* without *disconnecting or suppressing* them.

'Drag' on the pancreas Life-force energy (from pancreas trauma memory of suppressing our true feelings) weakens the emotional connections needed for us to connect with and discern our true feelings clearly and quickly, which causes us to feel depressed because of a disconnection from our true Self.

This drag that we 'take on' our pancreas Spirit Life-force allows us to survive by disconnecting in order to 'not feel' our true feelings. The trauma memory that creates pancreas issues comes from a history of enduring and suppressing our true feelings (because following and expressing our true feelings and divine intent didn't feel safe).

Disconnecting from following our pancreas Spirit's true feelings forces us to survive by *living in disconnection* from our true essence. This is not a sustainable, regenerative strategy and it will most likely lead to symptoms such as sugar or alcohol cravings, depression, pancreas health problems and pancreas emotional issues.

21. Posterior Pituitary Spirit Function - Our Rectifier

Our posterior pituitary Spirit Life-force energy gives us the ability to cleanse and free ourselves from getting stuck in the *grief of loss and the feelings of unworthiness.* Grieving hydrolyzes and cleanses our system with the power of water. These fluids in the form of tears were designed to wash us free from our losses. Our posterior pituitary energy allows us to cleanse our life by grieving over our losses (to free us from what is no more) to allow us to see our world anew, and to *accept our new reality.*

Posterior pituitary Spirit Life-force energy allows us to move into our new world *without* what *was,* and *with* what *is now.* This function is designed to release us from our *past* traumas of loss and allow us to be *free* to make the most of our present opportunities and abilities to create the future we desire.

The issue is about remaining stuck or becoming free from endless grief. This can only be done by consciously getting ahead of old unconscious memories of the way it 'use to be' – those habits that keep us stuck in thinking patterns about what was lost. A feeling of unworthiness can result in wondering what we could have done to 'save' that person we lost (if it was a death), or what we could have done to save the relationship of someone who is still living, etcetera). The effect of both of these situations turns out to be a feeling of loss and unworthiness.

These feelings are then often unconsciously projected into *current* feelings of *unworthiness* about our Self. I call it the *'could' a, would' a, should' a'* dragon, because of what we think we 'could' a, would' a, and should' a' done – but didn't do – causing us to remain feeling stuck in past times that can be no more (at a great cost to us in the long run).

Our power is in the moment and if we are in a time warp in our moments of power, we become stuck. And if we are in a loop of grief wondering what we could have done to change things 'back then', no wonder we unconsciously feel unworthy to live in the present! This creates justification to feel unworthy because it disconnects us to our present which is where worthiness is created. We cannot relive the present moment. Once it's gone, it's gone. This is why this dissociation creates such a heavy cost to our present because we cannot live in the present if we are *stuck in the past.*

Reversing these dysfunctional habits begins by *allowing ourselves to grieve* by following our posterior pituitary Spirit's responses to grieve, cleanse and accept our new reality in a timely manner that is free of our losses – *without just becoming stuck in our grief and loss.* Grieving requires sufficient consciousness to 'tune in' to our true feelings about our losses, and to then be able to feel safe enough to freely express our feelings of grief in an appropriate manner.

The posterior pituitary dragon enters the picture when our posterior pituitary Spirit Life-force energy gets programmed and conditioned by trauma memory of loss and 'not being enough.' This creates a 'drag' on freely expressing who we really are. At this point we become directed by our unconscious memory (of unworthiness and feelings of not being 'enough'). This effectively disconnects us from consciously recognizing Who we really are as Spirit beings because we are numb from being stuck in grief.

This keeps us feeling stuck in unresolved grief by stopping our posterior pituitary energy flow, spinning it backward, so that we defensively endure and survive 'not feeling' our devastating trauma of loss that settles into our feeling of unworthiness and 'not enough.'

This organ emotional trauma all boils down to the word 'without.' The dragon's solution is to *endure and survive 'being without.'* The posterior pituitary dragon's solution of *'surviving without'* perpetuates our 'feeling stuck' by feeling *unworthy of having* what our Spirit wants to fulfill our uniquely divine intent. (The symptoms of unresolved grief can appear as anger, guilt, disconnection and etc., but posterior pituitary drag usually relates to unworthy feelings from traumas of loss, or 'being without.')

Our posterior pituitary Spirit Life-force energy (of worthiness) always notices, either consciously or subconsciously when it is being ignored – even if it doesn't have the power to do anything about it. But if Spirit Life-force is flowing through the posterior pituitary circuits, feeling 'stuck' and 'not enough' is not a problem because Spirit keeps us 'in the know' of our infinite Self worth on a continual basis. And the nature of the posterior pituitary 'drag' is to *disconnect us from our feelings of worthiness.* And this loss and grief 'prison' will result in feelings of *negative self worth* on a continual basis.

In summary, this feeling of negative self worth makes us feel like we are *'not enough'* to deserve or have what our Spirit really wants. When this conditioning exists long enough it will physically manifest as body fluid imbalances (like dehydration and edema) along with an emotional feeling of being stuck. This feeling comes from unconsciously being *unable* to free ourselves from *thinking we have no choice* but to live 'without' and/or be 'not enough' (from rerunning old familiar associated memories of losses and living without having and being 'enough').

This enables a life of 'not enough' money, love, power, looks, and many other things, that prove to us (and make us feel and act 'as if') we are 'not enough' to deserve what our Spirit really wants. We may even be so we can't even think or talk about feeling and being worthy because it is so unimaginable!

The emotional function of the posterior pituitary is designed to allow us to feel and experience our own personal worthiness for just being Who we are as Spirit. We do this by feeling, knowing and being able to consciously get ahead of and separate ourselves from triggered past projections of old feelings of being 'unworthy.' On the other hand, the dragon needs us to believe the 'there is something wrong with you' scenario so it may own us. Because it continues to survive as long as it convinces us that we are not enough just being Who We Are.

We must be able to feel experience and project our own worthiness in order to be presently connected in our moments of power to create our best performances, which are needed to create the future we desire.

In other words, we need to have the emotional fine-tuning to consciously feel, discern, know and choose the differences between the *worth* of fulfilling our Spirit, and the *cost* of our 'drag.' Because the dragon strategy endures the distorted idea that we are *not-enough* and must *live without* and ignores our Spirit's true values by unconsciously choosing to be guided and directed by our dragons' defensive ways.

'Drag' on the posterior pituitary Life-force energy from our feeling memories of loss *diminishes our emotional ability to discern and feel the true worthiness of our Spirit's truth.* This drag on our posterior pituitary Spirit Life-force energy (which we take on to survive our traumas of loss and unworthiness) lessens our desire and ability to even try to be true to our Spirit Self. And then drag becomes a drag!

The conscious, elegant emotional solution for our posterior pituitary energy is to be able to consciously perceive and process our true worthiness, value and our grief from loss, to feel free and directed by our Spirit Self. Otherwise, we play the dragon's game of living our present through our projected past memories of *not enough* so we may endure and survive our familiar feelings of unworthiness as though we are *never going to be enough* to be accepted for just being Who We really Are as unlimited Spirit Beings. This thought is impossible to fathom because the posterior pituitary dragon just cannot get that concept, so it gets us to 'buy' the idea that we are far less than what we Really Are.

These feelings of *not enough* can lead to strange behaviors like hoarding things (because if we are never going to have enough, then we had better take everything we can get and hold onto it). Also, the word 'cheap' comes to mind (because if we are *not enough,* then we cannot even imagine being generous). The funny thing is, Reality spells out that there is nothing more valuable than accepting our True Worthiness and Personal Power that is of inestimable value!

In summary, the reactive trauma memory that creates posterior pituitary challenges and problems is a past history of having to endure traumas of loss and *not enough* that were never sufficiently processed. They never got 'hydrolyzed', or cried out, so the energy stays 'stuck.'

An example of how you might not be able to let go of the past is if you have thoughts about how you 'could' a, would' a, should' a' stopped the loss from happening somehow (even though it may have had nothing to do with you). The dragon thinks: "If you had been all that you **should have** been and done everything the way you **could have**, then that person **would not** have died. It's **all your fault** and because you are so unworthy, you need me so you can endure all this unworthiness!"

This leaves us with the feeling that no matter what we did, it was not enough and that's why that person died, etcetera. And since there is no resolution to this feeling, what takes over is the feeling of personal unworthiness (feelings of not *being enough*) that we cannot change or escape even onto our present.

And this is why God gave us the eleventh commandment: "Thou shalt not 'should on' one's Self!" ☺

Disconnection from our posterior pituitary Spirit's sense of true personal worth allows us to survive by living separated from our true Self that will be enacted as either a suppressed or perpetual, time warped 'grief loop' (making us feel unworthy either way). This is an unsustainable, degenerative strategy and over time can be associated with edema and/or dehydration (fluid balance) problems!

22. Parathyroid Spirit Function - Our Discerner

Our parathyroid Spirit Life-force energy gives us the natural ability to make refined discernment of differences to quickly and decisively separate what we *really want* from what we *really don't want.*

When it is necessary, this Spirit energy needs sufficient decisive intensity to break through and dissect the strong forces of rigid opposition that are up against our truth. So, this decisive energy is designed to give us sufficient strength to effectively and efficiently dissect and cut through external rigid opposition to our Spirit's truth.

The parathyroid Spirit Life-force energy gives us the ability to *decisively discern* what we *really do want* – from what we really *don't want.* This requires us to consciously stay ahead of our unconscious triggers from old habits of feeling unsafe being decisive about what we want. We can do this by being sufficiently decisive in our tone of voice to be believable enough in our expressions to clearly represent our truth about what we really *want* and what we really *don't want (by using our 'I mean it!' tone of voice).*

This first requires us to be able to consciously tune in to what we *do want.* And then we must feel safe to express our Spirit's real truth (about what our 'Spirit Self' sees, feels, wants, and does not want).

When we are programmed and directed by triggered, reactive and projected unconscious trauma memories of *not feeling safe being decisive about what we really want,* this causes us to be *indecisive* about what we want. When this happens, we tend to force our Self to *accept what we do not want,* which creates feelings of *anger* (the anger comes from *feeling forced to do* what we don't want to do, or to *not do* what we do want to do).

When we can consciously stay ahead of the drag of triggered memory (of indecisiveness causing us to not feel safe being and acting decisively true to our Self), we can then learn to decisively express what we want and don't want. And when we can do this in the appropriate tone of voice that clearly communicates what we truly *see, feel and want* (throat/parathyroid), our listeners have a better chance to really hear and know our truth because it is spoken so decisively that it is clearly expressed and leaves very little doubt about *what we really want!*

If we are *indecisive* in our *tone of voice* about *what we really want,* we are, in effect, emotionally communicating that what we *don't really want* is what we *really do want* which makes us really unbelievable! (In the movies this would be called a 'bad scene' and it won't sell tickets).

And since we are not believable, this invites others to tell us or help us decide what we want by telling us what they think we want. This may provoke our anger, but our parathyroid drag on Spirit Lifeforce suppresses our anger (which suppresses our decisiveness). This suppression keeps us feeling indecisive, so we reinforce what we don't want (which creates even more anger – which our dragon then suppresses). And either way, we never get what we want because we never show up for it!

This vicious cycle makes us resigned to feeling we have to do what we ***don't want to do***. This attracts others with dragons who want to control us. And if we are used to being controlled, we are (at first) naturally attracted to this familiar feeling like a 'match made it hell' (which this dragon attraction creates)! The trick is to recognize dragon energy by remembering the five words that describe it as well as to stay ahead of it. And again, those five words are: confusion, deception, manipulation, fear and force.

People who like to control us won't think twice about asking us to always do what they want us to with no thought being given to what we want (as though what we want doesn't really matter)! With all this going on, it's easy to see why *anger* is the emotion of the parathyroid.

Doing what we don't want to do can become so familiar that, over time, we just learn to *live indecisively* about everything we really do want or don't want just to avoid feeling clear and decisive enough to dissect the opposition. Otherwise we feel angry from not being decisive about what we really want. (This is what creates an attitude of: "Who cares?")

Anger is our system's 'last resort' energy for protecting us from being controlled by rigid oppositional forces. Scogna suggests that when anger over indecisive feelings is not expressed, the parathyroid actually stores our suppressed anger in calcium and deposits it (calcium production is one of the main functions of this organ, i.e. kidney stones) in the organ or gland where the drag is occurring.

These deposits help provide a physical resistance on the organ/ gland Spirit Life-force energy flow by blocking or slowing down what the organ is designed to do. For example, in organ number 16 (the kidney/filtering organ) the calcium deposit of anger is stored as kidney stones to give us enough 'hardened drag' to help resist expressing our Life-force energy function (kidney stones are calcium deposits resulting from not filtering toxic emotional situations, or what was not right emotionally for us).

The organ's emotional function reveals what's causing the problem in that organ (i.e., 'drag' on the parathyroid/kidney circuit means not expressing and resolving anger/decisiveness issues of not filtering out something that did not work for us emotionally). This is what is called the '16-22' uplink between these two organs – which is the blocked circuit between the parathyroid and kidney organ that is showing up in the kidney. The way it works is that the parathyroid is the organ that is *creating* the calcium deposit and the kidney is the one *receiving* it.

For instance, a secretary who hates her typing job but feels she has to do it for survival feels anger about feeling forced to type. Her body then may place calcium deposits (anger) in the precise place she is *doing* what she is *angry* about (in this case that would be in her *fingers* to help her stop typing). It can literally 'speak' this anger by calcifying and stiffening her fingers so she can't type!

The body is brilliant in how it attempts to emotionally communicate with us! The real question is: "Do we get the message that it is sending?"

The parathyroid dragon enters the picture when our parathyroid Life-force energy gets programmed and conditioned with 'drag' from traumas causing us to not feel safe being decisive about what we really want. So we take on the 'parathyroid dragon' which dims our perception for discriminating between what we really want and don't want (making us more indecisive about what we really want).

This spins our parathyroid energy backward to defensively endure and survive feeling forced to do what we don't want to do. We defend by being indecisive or when asked what we want, we say: "I don't know" instead of expressing what we really want. However, our Spirit always knows what we want, either consciously or semi-unconsciously – even if it does not have the power to act on it. But when parathyroid Spirit Life-force energy is flowing through our circuits, being indecisive is not a problem.

On the other hand, ignoring our Spirit's true desires creates our parathyroid *prison* of 'indecisive living' – which is rigidly living out of alignment with what our Spirit really wants.

The conscious elegant parathyroid Spirit solution is achieved by consciously using that decisive energy to perceive and follow our Spirit's truth. But playing the dragon's game distracts and diverts us from what we really want, by following our projected indecisive feelings from past memory, which is only one of the many ways we never get what we really want.

But there are other ways as well. For example, there is an old saying about the straight and narrow path that leads to happiness. It is a narrow path because it's always about staying in that perfect balance between the 'too much' or the 'too little' (which as we've discussed are both in dragon territory).

So, with that in mind, the other ways we can limit our ability to makes decisions includes the person who 'over-decides.' This is the person who wants to say 'yes' to all the 'decisions' placed before her. She actually 'over-decides' by liking and wanting to choose all of them and because of this can't make a decision about any of them! (Notice this ends up qualifying her as being indecisive which qualifies this as a parathyroid problem as well – because in the end, she wants them all but cannot pick any of them.)

In summary, the emotional function of the parathyroid energy is to perceive and express feeling differences that allow us to quickly know and say what we really want and what we really don't want. We do this emotionally by consciously feeling these differences that allow our feelings to instantly guide and direct us in our decisions/actions so they align with our Spirit's truth.

The 'drag' on our parathyroid Spirit Life-force energy flow weakens our desire and ability to be and stay true to our Spirit Self. (So drag creates the problem and then makes the problem worse over time.)

The un-cleared trauma memories that create parathyroid issues come from a history of having to *endure traumas of feeling unsafe to be decisive about what we really want.* This forces us to survive being separated from our Spirit's truth and we disconnect and do not follow our parathyroid Spirit Life-force energy. This defensive strategy is degenerative and unsustainable because it does not align with our Spirit ever being decisive about what it really wants. Being indecisive not only results in a 'drag' on parathyroid circuits, but often does it at the added expense of calcium deposits in 'telling' places.

23. Spleen Spirit Function - Our Rejecter

Our spleen Spirit Life-force energy provides us with the ability to *appreciate ourselves and others* by having enough self-respect to be able to *reject what antagonizes, disrespects or does not appreciate us.*

The function of our spleen Spirit Life-force energy is to 'remove us' by rejecting whatever and whoever is not respectful and appreciative of us. Spleen energy naturally rejects what antagonizes us (when it is without drag from trauma memory), which helps to better find who/ what does appreciate and respect us.

Spleen Spirit Life-force energy is designed to give us the ability to reject what antagonizes and disrespects us. This often requires the ability to consciously override old programmed habits of pleasing our antagonists (which reinforces, enables and maintains what antagonizes us).

Rejecting what antagonizes and disrespects us requires us first to have sufficient consciousness to consciously know when we are being respected and appreciated – and when we are being unappreciated and disrespected. Then, we must be willing and able to own and say, "This does not work for me!" and then observe who cares what works for you. This will indicate who appreciates you and who doesn't.

It is important for us to find out who respects us enough to care about what 'what works for us' – and who doesn't. Once we can do this effectively, we can better appreciate those who appreciate us quicker and be more able to reject those who disrespect us quicker. We can also 'get real' quicker with action in our body language that says we expect personal respect.

If our spleen Spirit Life-force energy is programmed by unconscious trauma memories of being rejected by those around us, we then reactively feel unappreciated by those around us. This causes us to reactively feel like we must please them to help assure ourselves that they care – and we must please them so that (just maybe) they won't reject us anymore if we do what they want!

Pleasing the antagonist contributes to allergic reactions because our body unconsciously tries to reject physically what we consciously refuse to reject emotionally. And instead of consciously rejecting what is antagonizing us, we reactively and unconsciously please those who are repeatedly disrespectful to us.

Our immune system can create physical allergic reactions when we are antagonized and do not reject what antagonizes us. Allergies are perpetuated by enduring longstanding feelings of being antagonized while trying to please others in order to feel more appreciated and less rejected. We do this to compensate for feeling unworthy of being appreciated. Of course this causes us to feel even more unappreciated and/or disrespected, so we need even more drag to endure these negative disrespectful feelings.

The *spleen dragon* enters the picture when our spleen Life-force energy flow is conditioned by the drag of trauma memory enduring feelings of being unsafe expressing spleen energy that rejects what does not appreciate or respect us. Spleen drag weakens our perceptual discernment for who does appreciate and respect us – and who does not.

Not rejecting those who disrespect and don't appreciate us can only happen by having a 'drag' on the spleen Spirit Life-force energy flow from the trauma memory of not feeling safe rejecting disrespect.

Our spleen dragon is designed to allow us to please our antagonisms, one day at a time. 'Drag' spins spleen energy backward to defensively endure and survive feeling disrespected and unappreciated from feeling unable to reject those who don't appreciate us (which our Spleen Life-force would do spontaneously without drag).

This often comes out in people who regret what they didn't do or wouldn't do or couldn't do because if they did, they would be following the spleen's Spirit which is to reject that which antagonizes you! This regret fuels the drag on the expression of rejection and perception of appreciation.

The spleen dragon's solution to disrespect from others is to please them and not notice the feelings of antagonism from disrespect. However, our Spirit always notices disrespect, either consciously or subconsciously – even if it doesn't have the power to do anything about it. But if Spirit Life-force energy is flowing through the spleen circuits, we won't have any problem noticing who disrespects us and figuring out what to do about it. And there will be very little regret (if any) involved because it feels good to respect our Self!

In summary, the emotional function of the spleen is to perceive the differences between feeling appreciated and respected – or not feeling appreciated or respected. In other words, we have the emotional ability to instantly and consciously feel respect and appreciation differences and use these feelings to guide and direct our daily path spontaneously through life. 'Drag' on our spleen Spirit Life-force energy weakens our emotional discrimination for consciously feeling the differences between feeling *respected* and feeling *disrespected* and/or unappreciated.

The drag on spleen Spirit Life-force energy that we take on to **not** reject what antagonizes us also allows us to endure and survive feeling unsafe rejecting what antagonizes us. This lessens our desire and ability to consciously be true to our spleen Spirit Life-force energy. Ignoring our spleen Spirit's truth feeds our spleen dragon to create a 'spleen prison' (living where we endure feeling disrespected and unappreciated – by enduring and surviving one day at a time).

The conscious, elegant emotional solution of our spleen Spirit Life-force energy instantly guides and directs us to reject disrespect and non-appreciation. This frees us from playing the dragon game of enduring disrespect and holding on to our regrets that maintain 'drag' on our ability to reject antagonism.

The triggered un-cleared trauma memories that create spleen issues come from a history of enduring feelings of it being unsafe to reject antagonistic disrespect. By not following (or acting on) our spleen Spirit Life-force energy, we become disconnected from it (which disconnects our spleen circuits). This forces us to survive by disrespecting our Spirit's truth. This is an unsustainable, degenerative strategy that will often lead to allergic reactions and spleen issues.

24. Lymph Spirit Function - Our Wizard

Lymph Spirit Life-force energy enables us to effectively *clarify the toxic mysteries of our Life* before our unsolved, misunderstood issues *cloud our understanding* and become harmful to our Life and health. It's about the choice to know and understand what energetic Reality is, or to not know and misunderstand what energetic Reality is.

The key to lymph Spirit energy is in knowing how to only accept what is acceptable and real. It is our 'inner knowing' (when we are Spirit connected in our circuits). To do this we must be like the wizard who knows the Ways of energy and instantly sees Reality clearly (through the Laws of energy) as what is *acceptable* and what is *not acceptable* because it doesn't work energetically. If our lymph circuits are flowing freely with Spirit Life-force, we will automatically 'know' (even if we do not act on our knowing).

If our lymph Spirit Life-force is blocked or disconnected, we may not realize we are missing something and may find ourselves 'living in mystery.' This is because we have been making our decisions by hunches that are energetically incorrect because they are not coming from Spirit Life-force Energy.

Our lymphatic Spirit Life-force energy system gives us the ability of the wizard who knows the Laws and Ways of how Spirit Life-force energy flows. This knowing detoxifies and clarifies the *energetic mysteries* of our life into *simple understandings* so we may see the *bigger picture beyond the senses* according to how things work energetically.

Continually being overwhelmed by feeling forced to *over-accept* what is *not acceptable* to our 'inner knowing' – creates addictive ways just to endure living in the mystery of *not knowing* and flowing with the ways of energetic Reality. If we do not see what is energetically Real because it is *inconvenient,* we may be tempted to cover this over with a quick fix. A quick fix can be anything from a simple 'happy face' to cover up *inconvenient truths,* to using hard drugs to escape Reality – or anything in between.

Lymph Spirit Life-force energy clarifies our understanding about the mysteries of who we are and how we function energetically, which allows us to consciously know what is real and what is not; effectively and spontaneously. This, in turn, gives us clarity to see how we need to perform in our moments of power to consciously stay ahead of our old habits of accepting toxic situations that are not acceptable. When we learn to do this, we are much more capable of making clear, quick, appropriate decisions that clarify what to accept and what not to accept into our life and/or body.

If it is allowed to decide, the lymph Spirit energy knows what is acceptable for the body's regeneration and what is not. Following our Spirit's clarity allows us to quickly avoid what is not acceptable/ degenerative by instantly and consciously tuning in to knowing our true feelings quickly for what *is* and *is not* acceptable to us and then being willing and able to act quickly in alignment with our Spirit truth according to what we know and feel.

If drag on our lymph Spirit Life-force energy is not consciously ahead of our unconscious reactive memory, the over acceptance function of the lymph dragon will make us feel that we need to accept unacceptable toxic situations in our life, and do it with a 'happy face.' This happy face might be covering up what we don't know *in order to be acceptable* to others. Or, it may be covering up our unwillingness to do what we do know. Either way, this fix might make everything feel and look great in the moment, but will devastate our life in the long run because of the continued drag on our lymph energy.

We are addictively drawn to quick fixes of relief to counterbalance the pressure of not being true to our truth. This drag to accomplish our fix creates the need for more drag to counterbalance that drag – hence the addiction to whatever that may be. We may spin our lymph energy backward to defensively endure and survive not being true to our Self by indiscriminate acceptance of what is unacceptable – counterbalanced by putting on a happy face, to make a show for the moment.

On the surface, these fixes make everything feel and look great, but devastate our life in the long run. Plus, doing this causes toxins to keep accumulating in our life and body because we fail to clarify them quickly enough by taking action to only accept what really works to regenerate our life and body.

In summary, the emotional function of the lymph is designed to perceive the *feeling differences* between *knowing what is acceptable to us and knowing what is not*. We are designed with the emotional ability to feel these differences and be consciously guided and directed by our Spirit's truth. Drag on the lymph Spirit Life-force energy clouds our emotional discernment for feeling what is acceptable to our inner knowing and what is not.

Our Spirit always notices what is and isn't acceptable – either consciously or subconsciously – even if we no longer have enough lymph power to do anything about it! But if lymph Spirit Life-force energy is flowing through our circuits, we will not only notice what is unacceptable, we will be clear about what needs to be done and truly happy to do something about it!

We take on an energetic 'drag' on our lymph energy flow in order to survive when we don't feel safe *discerning and expressing what isn't acceptable* to us. If we want to stay in denial of those inconvenient truths in our lives, we have to take on a lymph 'drag.' This 'drag' causes us to lose our inspiration for being true to our Spirit Self.

Ignoring our Spirit's truth creates our lymph energy 'prison' where we live in a world that is unacceptable to our Spirit in order to feel accepted by the outside world, by acting like it is acceptable! The lymph dragon's solution to such traumas is to first use a happy face to not notice and then accept what is unacceptable (followed by other quick fix addictions).

Failing to notice what is or isn't acceptable, and then counterbalancing our over acceptance of what is not acceptable with a 'happy face' is a drag on our lymph Life-force energy that serves to degenerate and dysfunction the very system that is designed to clarify our lives!

The elegant, emotional solution for our lymph energy is feeling safe and able to be consciously guided by our Spirit's truth about what kind of knowledge is or isn't acceptable (without playing the lymph dragon's game of over-accepting what is unacceptable to our inner knowing that is guided by Spirit).

Having a history of enduring traumas of feeling unsafe to see, feel or express what isn't acceptable creates these reactive trauma memories in the moment. Not connecting with and following our lymph Spirit's truth lessens the power of our lymph circuits, which forces us to survive by disconnecting from our lymph Spirit's truth, which keeps us in denial of our own inner knowing. This is an unsustainable, degenerative strategy that will lead to addictive dysfunctions and toxic lymph problems.

Chapter Summary

Our conditioned, unconscious reactive dragon patterns that are programmed into our organ/gland energy systems' memory are strengthened each time these patterns are repeated (as unconscious triggered reactive dragon habits). This also makes them more and more unconsciously controlled – the more they are repeated – until we *begin to identify with our dysfunctional patterns* as if they are 'us' instead of the 'not us' they really are. They become way too familiar and spontaneously performed *without the consciousness needed* for us to be able to get ahead of them and change them.

When our unconsciously programmed patterns are effective, productive and regenerative, this is great. But when our unconscious habit patterns are dysfunctional and degenerative they will continue to create ongoing degenerative programming (until we become conscious enough to change them in the moment of decision or power, where and when we are creating them).

Consciously knowing and choosing to live in the real world and accept what is real eliminates the 'drag' of fear and force in our lives. But the more we act out our dragon's defensive survival programming, the more we tend to identify with 'being' our dragon – by identifying with the dragon's behavior so much so that we think 'we are the dragon.' We will, in fact, define ourselves as 'being' our dragon's ways of surviving and enduring confusion, deception and manipulation, rather than knowing, following and identifying with our Spirit's Ways of Love and Light.

Once we identify with our dragons, we then tend to defend them and their needs and desires for their favorite drag (as if they were us). *When we feed the dragon, we perpetuate its programming,* even into the next generation, creating and supporting what I call 'the dragon's retirement plan.' That's because if we continue to follow our dragon's ways, we need more and more of the dragon's ways to continue – and around and around and around we go! By unconsciously repeating over and over again the same programmed, unconscious defensive decisions and actions, motivated by fear and confusion, we induce our children to unconsciously repeat the same decisions and actions!

We need to be conscious of what decisions/actions are needed to create the future we desire. However, in order to change these unconscious, automatic programs, we must be conscious in (or before) our moments of decision. And we will need to have sufficient perceptual clarity to make conscious discerning decisions and actions *before those moments are taken over by unconscious reactive memory.*

Consciousness allows us to make the subtle choices often needed to create health in our life and body and make us more capable of programming our decisions and actions to express our Spirit's Life-force energy. This becomes our power to effectively process and regenerate our life's *issues* – so they don't manifest as problems in the *tissues* of our body.

Consciousness is the only elegant solution!

Once we realize where, when and how we are expressing the 'drag' on our Life-force energy flow, we can *consciously* catch ourselves before our triggered memory reactivates old *unconscious* dragon decisions for us. At this point, we can consciously *imprint new decision-making patterns* and habits (with actual physical, synaptic changes from new learning). Our decisions and actions that follow this process will continue to update our memory banks with conscious, regenerative expressions that will direct our life more productively in our future.

> *Higher consciousness is having the ability to clearly and quickly perceive energetic Reality. This enables us to make clearer decisions that direct more effective performances and actions that align with our Spirit's Truth.*

If our Spirit Life-force energy is free to flow and consciously respond as designed through our magnificent system of *perceiving and expressing organ/gland energies* on multiple levels of functioning, then we have a naturally integrated and spontaneous ability to *prevent and resolve all our life and body problems* (that operate on different levels of energy).

Clear perceptions of energetic Reality followed by clear decisions that perform right actions with the right dose, at the right time – creates solutions and prevents or eliminates problems. As John Lennon said, in the lyrics to his song "Watching the Wheels," "There are no problems, only solutions."

With energetic Reality as our guide, our human potential is so much greater than what we have known since the 'fall' of conscious societies that may have known the secrets of the body's language encoded in the organs and glands and used them to ascend to levels of consciousness that were reflected in their writings.

Once we learn the language of the body – we too can open new doors to not only our health, but our longevity and fulfillment of our divine intent. And once we are living lives that are aligned with energetic Reality, we can see how a long life could be more possibly and be a much more attractive idea than living a life that is separated from any concept of how to really live it?

The next chapter sums up how this 'game of life' works energetically by using an actual infrared scan on a real client *and the organ/gland interpretation.*

KNOW THYSELF

Chapter 7

Case Study of Leyla, One of Dr. Allen's Clients

Leyla is a beautiful and successful Hollywood model and actress who began working with me in 2001. Her major complaint at the time was sugar cravings. As a model, this was considered a major problem and was not acceptable to her.

Her first infrared scan in 2001 revealed that her pancreas (20) was in her 'core,' acting as her dragon's 'subconscious coping strategy' (see her scan/chain below), which meant she was subconsciously programmed to cope with her problems by suppressing her true feelings.

Her cellular computer's programming code is revealed by her organ and gland energy scan and the output of numbers (what we call a 'chain') representing a sequenced code revealed from her infrared measurements. This feedback during our session showed Leyla her most significantly blocked electrical organ/gland energy flow circuits and patterns of her 253 circuits of personal Life-force energy providing her primary personal powers for dealing with and processing her daily life.

The infrared scan revealed her unique numerical chain that is her programming code for how she was presently living and making decisions in her life. I used this science to show her (in term of her own decisions and actions) where and how her 'operating system' is creating and maintaining defensive *homeostasis* in her life's decisions that are creating her problems.

These decisions and actions are her old familiar defensive ways of past memory instantly projected onto her present reality. This explained to her the facts regarding why she spontaneously *walked backward in her moments of truth* – instead of 'showing up' and *being true to her Self.*

This is the first step of consciousness, to clearly see *how we are creating our problem!*

[Remember there are two ways to create homeostatic balance. The first way creates homeostatic balance by using the Spiritual and natural Laws of energy. And the second way creates homeostatic balance by counterbalance; or, by counterbalancing the *present* 'drag' with the *past* 'drag' from our unconscious memories about how certain Life-force energies were conditioned to function in our past.]

Note: The following numbers (from 1 to 24) represent each of the organ and gland energy systems' *degenerative order* in terms of their importance for our *survival*. 1 represents the thymus, 2 is the heart, 3 is the colon, 4 is the stomach, and so on all the way up to the lymph (24) as listed in the previous chapter of this book. A reminder: the reason there are 23 organ systems and 24 numbers is because 17/18 is two numbers that represent the endocrine system. The reason for this is because the endocrine system functions on two basic levels of energy: the *etheric* and the *physical* to establish/maintain homeostasis.

Leyla's chain is listed many times in this chapter for the reader to follow the specific emotional dynamics involved in her various blocked circuits. We show Leyla's chain on each page for easy access so the reader can visually see energetically what is being explained in terms of her life.

This is Leyla's chain that describes her personal organ/gland energy sequences:

Leyla's Chain, for Reference
16 – <u>14</u> – <u>22</u> – 8 – <u>6</u> – **[20]** – <u>12</u> – 17/18 – <u>19</u> – <u>23</u> – **15**

We read Leyla's chain by beginning with her core organ, which is the one that falls in the middle position of her chain. Leyla's core organ is the pancreas (20), telling us that the 'drag' on her pancreas was functioning as an old, familiar *subconscious 'coping strategy'* by *dissociating her from her true feelings* and suppressing them. She did this so she could cope since she wasn't feeling safe and secure enough to express and follow her true feelings.

So, her core (20) 'drag' was her old familiar pancreas memory of subconscious habits of repeatedly *suppressing her true feelings* in order to please her father. This memory was used subconsciously to do the same thing in her present relationships that she learned to do in her past with her father (which was to cope by *suppressing her true feelings* because she did not feel safe being true to her Self). And when we met, she was still doing it because she did not *feel safe* thinking/acting like she deserved to get the sweetness her Spirit desires – or to even be *true to her feelings* and express her truth.

Such *coping behaviors* over time often manifested into pancreas issues (20) and problems like sugar cravings (Leyla's Major Complaint, or 'MC'). This integrated pattern was confirmed by (20) being in the core of Leyla's infrared scan/read-out (what is called her 'chain of numbers') that *matched* her physical symptom (sugar cravings), and her past father programming. So everything fit well in terms of connecting and integrating all of her dots ('20' in core of scan, sugar craving, past suppressive programming and current suppressive emotional behavior). This gave me validation that we were *connecting the real dots of her energetic Reality* and were on the right path to consciously *clear* her power-sucking problems so she could create her elegant solutions.

The pancreas (20) organ energy has the primary responsibility for processing sugar in our body and also perceiving and expressing our Spirit's true feelings. We need to find and follow these true feelings in order to manifest our divine intent. Our personal emotional powers of our pancreas energy are about our ability to feel safe perceiving and expressing our true feelings. Problems are created when we are motivated by the fear from past trauma memory that has conditioned us to not feel safe and worthy expressing our own true feelings.

Leyla's emotional situations with her family were centered on her father who ruled the family with a military attitude somewhat void of a real heartfelt connection that could relate to her sweetness and her true feelings. So she learned to suppress them. (This type of suppression actually *attracts* those who *would rather not be bothered* with us expressing our true feelings.)

Leyla's scan also told me that her *kidney* (16) *'drag'* was her lead counterbalance of her core pancreas 'drag' of coping by suppressing her true feelings (20). She counterbalanced this suppressive drag with an equal/opposite drag to suppress her kidney (16) energy (emotional filter) by not saying what didn't work for her emotionally. She didn't filter what didn't work for her emotionally because in order to maintain homeostasis she needed to counterbalance the drag on her pancreas (20) with a drag on her kidney (16). This was true for the obvious reason that if her defensive plan was to not express her true feelings (which didn't work for her emotionally), then she couldn't violate her own plan by filtering out what didn't work for her!

> ### Leyla's Chain, for further reference
> **16** – 14 – 22 – 8 – 6 – **[20]** – 12 – 17/18 – 19 – 23 – **15**

We can think of counterbalancing (to achieve homeostasis) as working like how a tightrope walker using a balance pole with equal opposing 'weight/drag' on each end of the pole to counterbalance, steady and hold his balance. For Leyla, a 'drag' on both organ energies created the equal and opposite drag needed to create the illusion of peace in the moment while living disconnected from her Self to achieve defensive homeostasis and maintain her Life-force energy with a short-term degenerative solution.

The obvious problem of using *drag* to create homeostasis is that the force is *backward* and *'down and in'* and *subtracts* our Life-force energy in order to accomplish short-term *degenerative* homeostasis. It is the short term solution with a long term problem – which is what the dragon is famous for!

Leyla was programmed to endure toxic emotional situations from not filtering (16/kidney issue) in order to counterbalance her programming of not expressing (suppressing) her true feelings (20/pancreas issue), in order to defensively create homeostasis by 'drag', which is quick, easy and *costly* long term.

However, since 'dragon' homeostatic balance is achieved by 'drag' *through counterbalancing,* that strategy is degenerative by nature and therefore unsustainable over time. This is because the dragon force used to achieve homeostasis by 'drag,' (the pulling magnetic force of trauma/fear memory by spinning our Life-force energy backward), creates *degeneration in the organs involved over time.*

In the case of Leyla, rather than expressing her true feelings (the 20/pancreas Spirit function) clearly, quickly, appropriately, and consciously ahead of the curve of electrical 'drag,' she had unconsciously over-learned to do the short-term degenerative solution.

And to make matters worse for the long run, she inadvertently learned to aid and abet the dragon by doing this defensive strategy more and more graciously (while learning to not notice the conflict) with better and better cover for her Spirit's truth until it broke down into the resulting long-term problems.

Our regenerative solution is always to achieve homeostasis through expression of our Spirit's truth by learning to express what Joe Scogna called: "The right dose at the right time." (Remember that optimal power is about effective performance within 1.1 seconds of the stimulus.) This enables us to show up clearly and to effectively walk the 'straight and narrow path' of energetic Reality to spontaneously claim our optimal personal power in those moments when it matters the *most*.

Leyla's Chain, for further reference

16 – 14 – 22 – 8 – 6 – **[20]** – 12 – 17/18 – 19 – 23 – **15**

The numbers/organs in Leyla's chain on the left, *between 16 and 20,* revealed her more conscious effect patterns that told her more *conscious story*. The numbers/organs on the right side, *between 20 and 15, gave* us the details for her more *unconscious story of cause* (identified by the patterns of decisions she was making early in life that conditioned/programmed her toxic emotional *effects*).

Over time, this therapeutic process has allowed her to become much more conscious of the bigger energetic picture of where, when, how and with whom these decision and actions have and do happen – to cause, enable and maintain her major complaints.

When Leyla suppressed her true feelings (with her 20/pancreas dragon) she had to then counterbalance her suppressed true feelings by also suppressing her desires (with her 6-liver dragon) to get what she really wanted. This allowed Leyla to defensively endure and survive not getting what she really wanted in the moment. But it led to her having sugar cravings (from not feeling safe to express her true feelings [sweetness] in her life), and cravings for more 'sweetness' to feel more safe and worthy of love.

Because of her emotional programming, Leyla's core dragon issue was around coping with the toxic emotional situations in her life because she was in a habit of not consciously noticing or being able to accept and express her true feelings so she could filter out (16-kidney) what did not work for her emotionally, which would purify her life. Otherwise, she was left with the defensive posture of *not* being true to her Self by taking on a kidney (16) 'drag' to help her to endure and survive the unfiltered toxic emotional situations in her energetic environment.

This unconscious dragon solution had caused Leyla to continue to create, maintain and endure her problem. This also prevented her from creating her elegant solution, which was to consciously perceive and express her truth clearly, quickly and appropriately (to see who cared about her true feelings).

Her dragons had always masked her true feelings, which kept her from connecting with the deeper levels of her true feelings (which can only be accessed and expressed by feeling safe and worthy of love.)

When Leyla finally learned to express more, she reported having fewer sugar cravings for 'sweet connections' (which resulted from her newfound ability to be more real with her Self and others). The cravings also lessened when she felt safer being more connected with her truth and able to express her true feelings better.

When Leyla's 'real' expressions of her true feelings were shut down, she became 'dragon bait.' This meant that she found herself accepting and even drawn to dragon-controlled men (who were *attracted to her not feeling safe and worthy enough to quickly know and express her true feelings*). This translated to her being more easily controlled by simply triggering whatever made her not feel safe (which is what the 'modus operandi' of the dragon energy is all about). See the problem so far?

Leyla's Chain, for further reference
16 – 14 – 22 – 8 – 6 – **[20]** – 12 – 17/18 – 19 – 23 – **15**

Conscious, elegant solutions always come down to first *perceiving* and knowing our truth clearly and quickly – and then being able to quickly *express* our truth clearly and appropriately. When we do this with a loving intent, a quest for the truth, a 'Mona Lisa' smile, and a great sense of humor, we can always create almost anything our Spirit really desires. (It also helps if we do not take things in life too personally or too seriously.)

Other insights from Leyla's chain

Leyla's chain also suggested that her indecisiveness (22/parathyroid) might be related to separation and disconnection issues in her relationships (8/sex organs). This could have been due to Leyla feeling unsafe transmuting (6/liver) her true feelings into her relationships (8/sex organs). The 6-20 (liver and pancreas) blocked circuit also indicated an inability to get what she wanted in her relationships (8/sex organs) by expressing her true feelings (20/pancreas).

To be in relationships, Leyla defensively separated and disconnected in order to feel safe, which allowed her to survive feeling unsafe in her relationships. This left her feeling like the sweetness was gone in her life because even though she was in a relationship she felt alone. (There is no 'alone' greater than the 'alone' of being with someone that you can't feel safe communicating with.)

This brings us back to Leyla's core issue (20) in a blocked circuit with the pancreas (6-20/liver- pancreas circuit). This created a 'drag' on transmuting her true feelings by first consciously disconnecting them from being clearly and quickly expressed freely and spontaneously in her relationships to finally have real connections with herself and her relationships (8/sex organs). Note the energy flow 'blocks' that are underlined in Leyla's chain that show where she counterbalanced her Life-force energy flow by using 'drag' for defensive homeostasis – which played out by not expressing her true feelings.

Reading a chain from right to left, we see what is going on energetically and how our unconscious causes (triggered reactive decisions) create our conscious effects (symptoms and problems). These all have messages about their powers that need to be fulfilled as problems or solutions (*if* we get the message).

Leyla's core (20) issue of coping by not really connecting with or expressing her truth with others allowed her to survive by suppressing her true perceptions – but when she suppresses, she can never see who really cares what she really feels, and who doesn't (because she never 'showed up' to find out). Doing this means she will never be able to transmute what she's got into what she wants (6/liver) because that requires expressing her true feelings (20/pancreas) consistently and effectively in order to create what her Spirit wants.

If Leyla couldn't feel safe being real spontaneously, she had to defensively cope in her relationships by re-enacting past memory in her present by repeating old patterns of not expressing her true feelings. This created the reactive unconscious defensive habit the American Indians call 'backward walking.' This is always the dragon's way of surviving 'one moment at a time.' But remember, *there are no points for defense in life or in any other game!*

In general, a chain shows our conscious *effects* and our unconscious *causes* from conditioned trauma memory patterns in our cellular computer. These memory patterns program our defensive dragon survival strategies that override and prevent our Spirit's offensive fulfillment which are the solutions to the challenges in our lives.

Leyla's Chain, for further reference
16 – 14 – 22 – 8 – 6 – **[20]** – 12 – 17/18 – 19 – 23 – **15**

The *left side* of all infrared scan chains reveals our conscious *effects* (or the symptomatic effects of our programmed decisions and actions of trauma memory). And the *right side* of the chain covers more of our unconscious programming with the subtle memory decisions of the prime *cause* which is called the *'anchor.'* (The anchor number in Leyla's case is 15/hypothalamus.)

The anchor serves as our *unconscious philosophy* about whether to show up and do what regenerates that organ or not (to 'be' or 'not to be') – based on that particular organ/gland decision. Using Shakespeare's idea once again, Leyla's anchor choice was 'to be' hypothalamus (which is to perceive and express the hypothalamus Life-force of sensory functions), or *not* 'to be' her hypothalamus Life-force energy function by tuning in to those circuits' functions.

Each decision we make is about 'being' or 'not being.' For all humans in general, it all boils down to decisions and actions that are *either* conscious and regenerative or unconscious and degenerative. This decision (made within one-thousandth of a second from the triggering stimulus) sets our prime cause organizing philosophy to follow either an *offensive* or *defensive* 'marching order' for the remaining down line organ/gland energy systems to follow to deal with our life's challenges.

Most people are more conscious of the organ issues as symptoms – which are closer to the *conscious effect* end of the chain (in this case the effect of the chain is 16/kidney). This is how and where our blocked circuits will eventually manifest into physical organ/gland symptoms after emotional and mental symptoms have existed for a sufficient time to manifest into this more dense physical energy!

Effect issues relate to the organ/gland scan numbers on the left side of the chain, which are our conscious *symptoms*. The left side of the chain is programmed by the right side unconscious asymptomatic (without symptoms) *cause* issues on the chain. These numbers reveal how our Spirit Life-force energy has been programmed by our trauma memory (the more etheric energy) to create specific emotional dys-functions that eventually, if and when repeated enough, will manifest into our *denser life problems* and *physical body symptoms.*

In summary, the organ/gland numbers on the right side of the core represent the *unconscious 'cause'* side of our programming code (the scan's chain of numbers) and the numbers on left side of the core rep-resent the *conscious 'effect'* side of our programming. The right side of the chain programs the left which represents how the unconscious causes (right) program the conscious effects (left). The center core number of our chain is our *subconscious coping strategy.* For Leyla, this was #20 (pancreas), indicating her old habit of suppressing her true feelings.

Leyla's first organ to the right of the core (in her chain above) was 12 (brain/nervous system), located in what is called the 'first cause' position of the chain. That organ issue is the *'first cause'* of her core 'coping strategy' (of suppressing her true feelings), because of her unconscious programming to endure and survive nervous confusions and complications (12/brain and nervous system) while 'walking on eggshells' (17/18/endocrine system) as gracefully as possible to avoid trauma by giving up her identity (19/skin) while being a pleaser (23/spleen).

Consequently, from that view, she probably felt her only choice (in the world where she lived emotionally) was to suppress her true feelings and not express herself (20/pancreas). (And she refined this strategy to make it look very good while she was doing it!) But her strategy was defensive so it was still degenerative to her Life-force over time (which results in aging).

She may have performed this defensive strategy too well as it turns out – because her endocrine-brain circuit was blocked (12-17/18). This shows us that Leyla's defensive strategy was to endure and survive the confusions and complications of the trauma in her life from feeling like she had to walk on eggshells to avoid short-term trauma (while creating long-term problems by living in a degenerative and defensive posture for too long and too well).

Leyla's Chain, for further reference
16 – 14 – 22 – 8 – 6 – **[20]** – 12 – 17/18 – 19 – 23 – **15**

If adopted on a long term basis, this strategy can easily become totally consuming of one's Life-force energy functions. This way of 'living' is consumed by 'living in trauma' – always trying to 'keep the peace' while 'walking on eggshells'! The endocrine system dragon loves this program (because survival is it's 'game'). The best result that can come from this is to survive and endure living in trauma *as if* we had no other choice. But this decision degenerates our Life-force over time.

The organ to the right of 17/18 (endocrine system), number (19), told me what was causing Leyla to endure living in trauma. For her, it was her skin issue (19), whose energetic function is to *define, defend and express* her true Self/identity. A 'drag' on the endocrine/skin dragon (17/18-19) is all about enduring and surviving without identity by *not* defining, defending and expressing one's true Self.

So a feeling of lost identity is apparently what set Leyla up for having to *walk on eggshells* as indicated by the numbers (17/18-19) in her chain. The spleen (23) Spirit energy's job is to reject what does not appreciate or respect us. However, the spleen dragon issue is all about *enduring and surviving* those who disrespect us and do not appreciate us (because we must please and endure antagonisms if we do *not* reject them).

Leyla was unconsciously programmed to feel traumatized (17/18/endocrine system) about expressing her true identity (19/skin) because she was programmed to please the antagonists (23/spleen) and not reject them – which caused her to not feel safe rejecting (23) those who didn't respect or appreciate (23) her.

This meant she had to re-program and discipline her dragons to 'be' and act consciously (a big job for her since her dragons continually wanted *get by with and put up with* continuous disrespect and lack of appreciation for her). However, no real connection was even possible in her future if this energy could not turned around first!

Now, finally, we come to the unconscious *prime cause* position of Leyla's chain/programming that made her first unconscious decisions (within a 1000th of a second of any triggered stimuli), for her 'to *be* or *not be*' the Spirit Life-force energy function of her last organ (15/ hypothalamus) in her chain

Leyla's Chain, for further reference
16 – 14 – 22 – 8 – 6 – **[20]** – 12 – 17/18 – 19 – 23 – **15**

The last organ number/function in Leyla's chain was her hypothalamus (15), which is designed to provide Leyla with the unconscious philosophy that directs the other organ/gland energies to act either proactively (to be) or reactively (to not be) to comply with her anchor *defensive* or *offensive* philosophy (15).

This last position number/organ is the unconscious 'prime cause' memory *that makes that critical first decision – to be, or not to be.* For Leyla, it is the hypothalamus. This is where her processing all began within a 1/1000/sec from any stimulus that ever called for a decision in her life!

We call this anchor position the 'prime cause' because it is our first unconscious decision (in a sequence of decisions); and if this first unconscious decision is defensive in nature (to 'not be' what the organ is designed to do) – it will degenerate Spirit Life-force as a series of continuous defensive decisions that will manifest as denser and denser energy problems.

Dragon patterns have a tendency to repeat (due to the dragon's unwillingness to change), and this is why these defensive decisions will result in larger life problems as well as physical symptoms if that behavior persists over time. Now can you see how the left side of the chain is a result of the right side and how prime cause philosophy governs the entire sequence of events that are creating problems in Leyla's life?

Defensive 'first decisions' are like telling a lie. The *first lie* requires us to support it with *another lie,* and then another lie, etc., because that first decision (that must be made) is a philosophical decision that sets our direction for either 'being or not being' true to our truth – a decision that must be made almost instantly in order to know and direct *how* we are going to approach each daily challenge we face.

"If we don't stand for something, we could fall for anything," goes the old saying. Pretty soon we forget what our truth really is, because it is buried under so many lies! It works the same way when we don't tune in to our truth continuously and listen to the subtle promptings of our Spirit. We then set ourselves up for one problem after another to mentally, emotionally and physically get ourselves off balance.

For Leyla the question was 'to be or not to be' hypothalamus (15). To 'be', she needed to clearly tune in to and attend to what her senses and feelings were *telling her*, and then she needed to be *willing and able* to communicate her truth clearly quickly and appropriately to create the results she desired. If not, her hypothalamus dragon fear would control her decisions and cause her to 'not be' hypothalamus (which is about being clear about what she senses). This would leave her feeling unsafe sensing or communicating – so she would unconsciously choose to defensively to endure and survive by *inhibiting her sensing and communicating.*

Leyla's Chain, for further reference
16 – 14 – 22 – 8 – 6 – **[20]** – 12 – 17/18 – 19 – 23 – **15**

In order to change her defensive unconscious philosophy, Leyla needed to become aware of when, where, how and with whom she did this daily. Then she needed to recall specific 'scenes' from her life's movie, where in the past she followed this defensive behavior pattern. And in her moments of power she had to imagine being able to connect with her senses spontaneously, and feel safe communicating her truth.

Her therapeutic assignment I gave her was to mentally re-script those scenes in her imagery using an *offensive hypothalamus philosophy* of being connected to her senses and by clearly communicating what she sensed so she could create the results she wanted in her life. I knew that if she couldn't feel safe doing that – then maybe this gut feeling might have been telling her that this was a degenerative pattern and that she couldn't continue to 'be' where she did not feel safe being true to her Self. (This is generally true for everyone, because as time goes on, more and more energy can get gobbled up into trying to look good even when we don't feel good about what is going on in our lives!)

The process of re-scripting *bad scenes into great scenes* allowed Leyla to first become aware of how she was creating her problems. It stimulated her consciousness by turning her unconscious dysfunctional pattern into more functional communication while she learned to consciously express what she sensed and felt while she was processing.

It is important to note here how unconscious the dragon really is. It lives in a 'cave' and is blind, after all! The hypothalamus' (15) dragon actually wants to **protect** Leyla. In the dragon's mind, it is always trying to protect us and help us survive, but since this energy is the blind master of darkness (unconsciousness), it can only provide short-term solutions that have long term problems.

So the dragon tries to protect Leyla by processing whatever it perceives through its limited logic and perceptions (which is its old defensive programming idea). Its philosophy is: "Since we must inhibit what we communicate and what we sense, how then is the best way to process what we see, hear, taste, touch, and smell *without communicating our real truth?*" Can you see how this idea means no hope for real solutions? (Note: The "Since you must" idea is the dragon's twist that time-warp's this *past unconscious assumption* into our present by literally thinking backward from how things really are in the present!)

With this defensive logic operating unconsciously, Leyla's first decision is to 'not be' true to her hypothalamus Spirit's power for clear sensory perceptions and communication (when she needs to do that the most). Instead, she projects past memory of how she had to deal with her father. She spontaneously and unconsciously chooses familiar short-term solutions which begin by first dissociating from what she senses, and then screening and inhibiting her *communication* about what she feels.

Sometimes we may need such a short-term strategy when we have no other choice and need to survive what we cannot change or escape (like when we are in childhood or in prison). But as a general rule, *if* we really *do need* to be in defense, we need to not be 'where we are.' And the only thing that works for our Spirit in that situation is an *'exit strategy.'*

If we really don't need to be in defense, we must consciously get ahead of reactively being in defense or going into defense, because it wastes our time and energy while it degenerates our regenerative Lifeforce energy (so we lose the strength of our personal power).

Leyla's Chain, for further reference

16 – 14 – 22 – 8 – 6 – **[20]** – 12 – 17/18 – 19 – 23 – **15**

And, if we live in defense (and we're *not* in childhood or prison), *then we create our very own prison around us* by following a defensive strategy that disconnects us from our Self and everyone else!

The reason our unconscious 'prime cause' *anchor decision is so important* – is because it sets our direction for either following the conscious regenerative ways of our Spirit, or for following the defensive unconscious degenerative ways of the dragon.

These boil down to following either *sustainable* strategies based on the regenerative solution-oriented Ways of our Spirit, or the *unsustainable*, degenerative, defensive, survival-oriented ways of the dragon.

Our hypothalamus (15) processes all sensory input and is designed to allow us to focus our attention on what our Spirit wants and needs to focus on at the right time.

If our senses are traumatized into focusing on what we need to survive (so we are not able to focus our senses on what our Spirit desires), the effect may be to defensively either *over-attend* or *under-attend* to what is needed.

When Leyla inhibits her natural ability to focus and attend to what her hypothalamus Spirit Life-force energy senses are telling her, she may counterbalance this by attending (15/hypothalamus) to what pleases (23/spleen) others in the outside world to distract her from what she is sensing and feeling that her inside world needs to communicate. That's why we call the Spleen dragon (23) *'the pleaser.'*

In other words, even though her father was no longer present in her daily life, she found herself acting in the *same dysfunctional way as she did then when he was around in her childhood!*

She is now seeing how she is continuing to project this same 'pleaser' type of behavior onto many others currently in her life at the expense of her own Spirit, which enables behavior she does not really want.

Leyla's Chain, for further reference
16 – 14 – 22 – 8 – 6 – [20] – 12 – 17/18 – 19 – 23 – 15

Through our work together, Leyla has become much more conscious of these issues and how they relate to her relationships with men (especially in her primary relationship), where she often unconsciously runs her old defensive programs of *reactively conforming* with external demands when she internally disagrees with them.

Then, as long as she could emotionally separate and disconnect *(8/sex organs)* from her true feelings (20/pancreas), she could have a disconnected relationship by learning to endure not feeling safe being real while trying to have a real connected relationship – which couldn't work 'then' or 'now.'

Because of this work, at present – Leyla is much more in touch with her truth. Instead of disconnecting from it and being directed by whatever somebody else wants, she can not only see how she has lost her power in the past, but is much more willing to do something about it in the present.

According to Leyla's more recent scans, she has become more conscious of how and when she separates and disconnects in her relationships with men, and she has also become much more conscious of where, when and how she is suppressing authentic expressions of her true feelings.

Anyone who knows Leyla has seen her become more conscious in her expressions. There has been a noticeable change in how she expresses herself more clearly, quickly and appropriately being aligned with her truth, than she did before by becoming more conscious from doing her work. But when she forgets to follow her new learning, she reports that her sugar cravings come back. However, what she now knows is that she is just a *conscious decision* away from turning the direction of her Spirit energy 'north' again toward rejuvenation and regeneration of every cell in her body.

Her defensive programming was very functional for following her father's rules when she was a child, in situations where she had no power and was not able to control, change or escape that dependent situation. But if she can continue to choose a more rejuvenative and pro-active agenda – her choices will lead her to the 'sweetness' in life she has always wanted.

KNOW THYSELF

The Summary and Conclusion

Psychology as the Subtle Energy Science of Consciousness

The science and field of psychology began with William James, who clearly saw psychology as being *all about consciousness!* However, James's perspective was soon usurped by the *behaviorist mentality* that provided a *denser* and more obvious level of scientific measurement. This approach, unfortunately, reduced psychology to being viewed as a denser energy science rather than the subtle energy science of consciousness that William James clearly saw. He held a bigger picture view of how psychology is about consciousness for the most evolved aspects of who we are at our most refined levels of functioning.

This *behaviorist takeover* did allow psychology to become more accepted at that time, because gross behavioral measurements allowed psychology to look more like the popular physiological sciences oriented around dense energy symptomatic effects (the medical model). This symptomatic effect-oriented model was well on its way to becoming an established and accepted idea for human health care by the late 1800's, accepted by nearly all medical authorities.

However, effect-oriented healthcare is only capable of providing short-term symptomatic care (often for the effects of our unconscious subtle trauma memory programming that creates most human problems) – with no attention on our problem's subtle-energy messages that reveal our most elegant solutions.

A hundred years ago, having a symptomatic effect-oriented behavioral philosophy may have been convenient, given how the popular view of the times was focused on our denser energetic reality that we can see in the visible spectrum of energy. However, the very nature and essence of psychology (as William James made clear) is mostly about subtle energetic Reality experiences of (i.e. organ/gland consciousness and trauma memory) that don't exist in the 3rd dimensional visible spectrum of energetic Reality. Rather, they exist in the 4th dimensional energy of time as programmed memory from our past.

Psychology is the subtle-energy science designed to scientifically integrate human energetic functioning to light the path for evolving humans to see how our consciousness directly relates to our health and fulfillment. Infrared science provides a significant contribution that allows us to scientifically observe and individually decode the *effects* of trauma memory and how they mentally, emotionally, and unconsciously program our organ/gland energetic tools that provide our perceptions and expressions.

Infrared science can now finally provide a subtle-energy science of psychology that integrates with our biology and subtle-energy physics of memory to incorporate a functional view of human consciousness that aligns with William James's original conceptions of psychology being a 'science of consciousness.'

Infrared science now maps out how we humans are designed to function as whole integrated energy systems of personal power. It also shows us how we 'come to' dysfunction from unconscious drag that disintegrates our conscious functioning with triggered and projected unconscious trauma memory. And, finally it shows us how to decode our symptoms' messages into our elegant solutions that allow us to consciously program our Life-force energy in order to fulfill our lives with our divine intent.

With infrared science, psychology can now reveal how our 'drag' on subtle organ/gland energy flow is programmed by past triggered memory that unconsciously makes our decisions and directs our actions.

We can now see how these unconscious issues block our ability to effectively get ahead of and solve all human problems by causing us to hesitate or not 'show up' in the moment. It shows us how rejuvenation results from each organ/gland's emotional perception being appropriately expressed (as long as we are consciously connected to the organ/gland's Spirit Life-force energy).

In Joseph Scogna's dichotomy work (*The Secret of SAF,* 1987), he defines psychology as being the science that *tracks unconscious memory* into *conscious experiences.* I have used infrared science with thousands of clients over the past twenty-five years and can verify that this method clearly shows how our unconscious memory can be tracked into our conscious experiences. [For a better description of this process in my clients' own words, see my 'Clients' Feedback' section on my website, http://dgallenphd.com]

Just like the Rosetta Stone clearly translated coded languages into coherent connections, our organ/gland energy-motion (emotional) language (with infrared science) decodes our Spirit's Life-force energy flow patterns into consciousness for real and elegant solutions to personal human life and body problems.

If we *cannot* decode these messages, then we *will* continue to create deeper problems that manifest into denser symptoms in our life and body. And these dense *issues* will eventually manifest into our *tissues* so our daily problems become harder and harder to resolve or deal with effectively and productively!

With infrared science and our organ/gland language to measure and decode our subtle energy flow patterns, we can now effectively provide cause-oriented solutions to our personal health problems as well as the more subtle 'psychological' health problems that confuse humans in dealing with their daily lives.

Psychology can now track/decode these personal subtle energy flow patterns into our personal "Ah ha's!" These energy patterns are decoded by natural organic insights to reveal how our Spirit Life-force energy flow is blocked by trauma memory 'drag' disintegrating our mental, emotional and physical functioning.

Consciousness is the Only Real Solution to Human Problems

Enlightenment is consciousness in action at the speed of light! And when it flows continuously, or equal to the speed we are receiving input – we can stay conscious of our input processing. This is how true higher consciousness happens spontaneously and continuously in-the-moment and when implemented can create conscious actions directed by the Love and Light that clarifies God's subtle Laws and Ways of energetic Reality so we can 'be here now' and be at peace with our Self.

For example, to be visually conscious, everything we see through our eyes must be processed at the speed of light for us to stay conscious of our visual input as it is happening. In other words, how many frames per second (FPS) are we processing consciously clear? The fact is that our personal power is primarily determined by the quality and speed at which we are able to consciously process our input into decisions that produce effective actions in our moments of power immediately following the stimulus!

If the way things really are *(Big 'R' Reality)* does not conceptually align with the hypothetical way we 'think' things are (little 'r' reality), then our confused conception of that reality will create conflicts between our mind's eye vision of the world, and the world that actually exists as energetic Reality. This conflict will inevitably create symptoms with messages that will prevent the problem and tell us how to create the elegant solution for that problem IF we get the message and follow it.

So our ability to conceptualize' energetic Reality accurately determines our ability to process Reality as it actually exists, which is required to be able to, direct and perform effectively in the 'movie' of our life.

To be *con-fused* is to believe in a 'con' about *'fusion'* (or how it all comes together that is not true). And if our ability to conceptualize Reality is confused and/or incomplete, or distorted, our concepts cannot 'fuse' with energetic Reality – and our life's 'movie' won't sell tickets!

To be effective, we must perform our truth by walking the straight and narrow path of refined energetic Reality by continuously balancing clear perception and expression (avoiding too much and not enough) with the right dose at the right time. This is how we begin to see and live the bigger, more subtle picture of Reality beyond the rainbow of 'physicality' to learn to walk on the edge of enlightenment, to immediately process our emotional energies so we can finally bring everything together into a fusion of energetic Reality as *One* whole, quantum dynamic, cosmic connection of energetic understanding.

Summary of the Ways of Energy

The 'Ways of our Spirit' feel good to us because they spontaneously connect us with who we are and what we see and feel and then align that with what we say and do in how we express our truth, with those who are safe and trustworthy to respect our Spirit and appreciate our process of living life.

Following our Spirit Ways of being consciously connected to knowing and acting out Who We Really Are energetically allows us to spontaneously perform these Ways of consciousness so we are continually spinning our energy 'up and out,' which regenerates our Life-force and rejuvenates our Soul.

The 'ways of the dragon' feel 'bad' to our Spirit (but feel 'good' to the dragon). This is because dragons are designed to survive traumatic perversions by disconnecting from energetic Reality. This disconnects us from our true feelings to not consciously 'feel so bad' when 'doing, seeing or feeling bad things.' Our dragons are in fact designed to disconnect us from our Spirit's natural feelings of connections with our twenty-three Spirit Life-force energies and their 253 circuits of personal powers (and problems).

The ways of the dragon naturally suppress the Ways of our Spirit Life-force energy in order to reactively endure and survive our present by using unconscious trauma memory programming to defensively do now what we had to do then for immediate survival.

This provides short-term homeostasis (solutions), but creates long-term degeneration (problems). The short-term solutions create the long-term problems of personal disease, disorder, dysfunction and degeneration that are mostly created by some type of defensive overreacting! This is a problem, because we can't regenerate when we are degenerating!

Consciousness is the only elegant solution because it is the only thing that gives us a conscious choice to know and create our real solutions. Otherwise, without consciousness, we unconsciously recreate our problems energetically by repeating reactive, short-term, dragon 'solutions' that reproduce themselves.

Consciousness allows us to have a conscious choice to express our Spirit's truth clearly, quickly and appropriately to be more effective and productive at claiming and performing our Spirit's personal power!

Dragon strategy is designed to defend us from what we *don't want,* and our ***Spirit strategy*** is designed to provide us with what we *do want!*

Since the Law of creation is: "What we focus on is what we create," it is most productive to focus on genuinely positive behavior characteristics (like those found in highly accomplished people) in order for us to learn how to create what our Spirit wants.

Abraham Maslow provided us with a great example of this approach after spending his entire career identifying actualizing characteristics commonly shared by highly productive and self-made people.

Common characteristics observed in highly actualized people can serve as our 'philosophical guide' to model and direct us toward more conscious decisions and actions in our life. Being aware of what 'actualized characteristics' really are and how they compare with our own behavior, can help us to recognize in ourselves in terms of what does, and does not align with sustainable evolved consciousness.

What we see in modern times is that usually the most successful people in any field are those who consistently make clear, quick, effective decisions and actions. How quickly and clearly they perform their truth, consistently, manifests as their success. This level of performance is needed in order for us to provide our most effective solutions for almost anything we do.

Stockbrokers who are successful give us an obvious example of how this principle of *timing* works, because success here only comes from being able to deliver the *right dose of the right thing in the right way at the right time.* In the stock market, timing is especially critical, since exact 'timing is what creates the most money' for the broker.

Winners are usually those who are most consistently clear, quick and appropriate over time. So, in the end, 'time will always tell' who are the most real, consistent and sustainable winners!

What allows everything to flow smoothly for everyone is for all of us to become conscious of energetic Reality (Source Energy's perfect plan of Laws and Ways) so we may all consciously learn to align with and follow these Rules, Ways and Laws of energy that define our most basic 'Reality.'

To do this we must integrate our understanding of Who We Are and evolve our consciousness so we may live consciously in alignment with energetic Reality. In other words, we need to make conscious decisions and take conscious *actions* that align with these Laws and Ways of physical, emotional, mental and Spirit Life-force energy functioning, in order to regenerate them and not degenerate them.

The higher our consciousness, the more naturally and quickly we are able to align our decisions and actions with the Way things already are energetically so they can work with energetic Reality. This eliminates and prevents all of our conflicts, which come from our lack of alignment with Reality!

All humans are made up of 253 circuits that are either partially blocked or flowing through our 23 organs and glands. And solving these organ/gland problems creates a sustainable nurturing environment for the whole of our life. I can't think of any problems that higher consciousness and alignment do not eventually solve. Since you are a human being with 253 circuits, higher consciousness (when used) has the potential to solve all problems in your health, in your business, and in your relationships.

To claim the full extent of our personal power in our moments of power, we must be able to clearly and quickly process our life experiences, through our various organs, at the speed of light. Events in our world are now moving faster and faster every day – as our 'quickening' into a conscious new world proceeds!

Seeing Our Problems as Messages About Our Undiscovered Solutions!

Energetic Reality seen with conscious clarity in the moment is the only thing that provides real and elegant solutions to all human problems because it is the only thing that gives us a conscious 'choice' to choose our Spirit's enlightened Ways, which allows us to perform so we can regenerate and rejuvenate here and now!

Problems are disguised opportunities for solutions. If we solve them, we can learn to achieve and manifest our Spirit's divine intent. This is the game that all humans play and it is a game that we are designed to win! It's just a matter of looking for the 'undiscovered solution,' because with clients *I have always found it to be there*.

The descriptive Laws of energy (physics and metaphysics) tell us exactly what and how we can manifest anything. Take the case of our symptoms: they are obviously simply feedback messages telling us what the problem is. When clearly perceived and understood, these messages reveal our elegant solutions, which can eliminate our problems *if* we make the decisions and take actions that create those solutions.

Fear is the emotion of the dragon that controls the sympathetic 'fight or flight' branch of our autonomic nervous system. Feelings of fear are at the heart of all stress and degeneration problems and issues!

President Roosevelt got it right, energetically, when he said, "We have nothing to fear – but fear itself."

Einstein had it energetically 'right' when he said: "Insanity: doing the same thing over and over again and expecting different results." The bottom line to all our discussions about energy is that continuing to unconsciously follow the ways of the dragon while expecting anything but long-term degeneration, is *delusional*, by definition.

Like I said before, today, it's all about getting the truth 'together' (like the 'hippies' said, "Get it together, man!" and 'Get real'). This turns out to be profoundly 'right on,' because the very first step in our personal evolvement of consciousness is to be able to 'get real' with the energetic Realities of our lives.

This also turns out to be also equally profound and simple, because our evolvement depends on our ability to 'get' our input (what we *see and feel*) 'together' and aligned with our output (what we *say* and *do*). These four memory functions of the four lobes of our cerebral cortex are what allow us to 'have it together' energetically so we can 'get Real' about Who We Are and how we function.

In my four decades of untangling this science of psycho-biophysics so I could learn how to integrate all my clients' energetic levels of their human functioning together, *infrared measurement* is the *only science* I have seen that is scientifically capable of *integrating* our entire human *physical, emotional and mental* programming of our Spirit Life-force energy into *one whole functional picture of our human system.*

Having a clear, scientific way to actually *track and see* how Life-force energy works in terms of when and where our 'drag' exists in our consciousness for our personal power, allows us to 'get it together' with *clearer decisions, more quickly.* This allows us to consciously align with the Ways and Laws of energetic Reality so we may consciously change the dysfunctional course of how we live our daily lives.

In working with this infrared science since 1987 to track and decode thousands of clients' electrical energy flow patterns from their body's own language of twenty-three systems and 253 organ/gland Life-force energy circuits; I have repeatedly marveled at the exquisite integration and profound wisdom consistently revealed from decoding the natural energetic flow functions of our physical, emotional, mental and Spirit Life-force organ/gland energies.

SUMMARY AND CONCLUSION

Tracking our body's energy flow patterns and decoding them with its own organ/gland language makes it abundantly clear that when we replace decisions and actions that *don't work* energetically (those that are degenerative) – with decisions and actions that *do work* energetically (those that are regenerative) – we replace our old world of problems with a new world that is much more personally functional.

Speaking of the 'old world,' anciently, secrets were passed down in arcane societies involving knowledge concerning *ley lines* – those latitudinal and longitudinal energetic lines that crisscross the earth holding magnetic currents that affected how electricity worked on the planet. This information affected almost everything in the outside world including their sea voyages, the planting of crops, and for our purposes in this book, was key to understanding how our bodies handle electricity as well!

King Solomon, the ancient Egyptians, and even purportedly those from Atlantis held these secrets about how things work and hid them in plain sight in the buildings they built with precise measurements that matched these ley lines of energy and keys that affected not only this earth but were intertwined with what measurements connected them to the cosmos. As my mother Elsie said: "Time will tell" about all of this, but what is so interesting to me is that some of the keepers of these secrets down through the ages actually identified themselves as dragons!

I am supposing that they were identifying with the 'dragons' that were the disciplined and evolved or the 'dragons in the sky' (those that had finally learned to yield and align their powers with Spirit Life-force energy so 'things could work' regeneratively).

In a book by Henrietta Bernstein, *Ark of the Covenant, Holy Grail: Message For The New Millennium* (DeVorss & Co., Marina del Ray, 1998, pp. 147-48), she capsulizes the Dragon story as follows:

"...the Dragons were a group of people who looked forward to a more harmonious way of life which they wanted to establish in America. They derived their name from the Druids, who were also called "Dragons" – those who knew how to control the ley lines of energy, often called the 'Dragon lines' of the geodetic earth currents."

243

They had heard about Atlantis and times before the 'fall of consciousness' and wanted to find and create a *new world* that included those high ideals for society that included consciousness. Many of them were considered rebels and heretics who wanted to find the new lands so they could migrate there to find the peace that their religions and politics could not provide them.

This illustrious group included many well known people that always seemed to be interested in furthering the Spiritual work on the planet. Some of them were burned at stakes and tortured in other ways simply for revealing inconvenient scientific truths that were not popular at the time. Some of them were world leaders that could never reveal how they really felt about the way things were in the societies they lived in. All of them contributed greatly to the knowledge base on the planet.

Many of these people had a passion to figure out the connection between 'true religion' and 'science.' They searched through books for information from ancient times that had not been 'skewed' by greed and ignorance. For many, the most they could hope for was a quest for 'true science' (that which followed the Spiritual and natural Laws of energy).

They mined and stashed gold and were obsessed with maps and compasses. They used these arks, boats, maps and ancient manuscripts to navigate their way to a 'new world' so they could establish a peaceful kingdom, a 'promised land' here on earth where freedom to 'be' was allowed. King Solomon and many others called these things the 'keys to the kingdom.' It was always a daunting task for sure, but something that they never ceased to want to accomplish for future generations!

I am both excited and humbled to share the profound insights that the long lost Language of our Body reveals. This truth has always been there for us to see for ourselves when we finally come to look at it from an energetic point of view. It is where science and true Spirituality 'come together' since this 'straight and narrow path' of energy is and has always been the 'key' to making things work in our lives!

And isn't it interesting that we have always had no further to look for these sacred secrets than the ley lines of energy in the ***body itself! They were inside of us all along*** where the organs and glands (which are 100% of Who We Are) quietly hid the secrets of not only our Divine Birthright as Spirits, but how that also directly connects our inner to our outer world and above to below as true *'Keys of the Kingdom.'* The answers were always there by 'Divine Design.'

As our world is evolving from the darkness to the Light – the time is *now* to recognize these rejuvenative 'clues' about our Self and begin to use them. This is how we can create real Spirit 'win-win' solutions to all our human problems! Because decisions made that rejuvenate from within the energetic ley lines and parameters of the Spiritual and natural laws of energy of each organ/gland energy system are naturally and directly reflected in our outer world. When you live life the way it works – it works!

When I was young, I could not have imagined the world we are living today, not to mention what we see coming for tomorrow. Today we have many choices before us that can create a better, more conscious world, motivated and directed by clarity and Love instead of by fear and confusion.

Living in a conscious world requires us to authentically and proactively express our truth clearly, quickly and appropriately in order to be able to fulfill our divine intent. Continuing to defensively suppress our truth (creating dysfunction and degeneration) in order to endure and survive one day at a time in fear and confusion – is no longer a viable option if we want to evolve and even survive the new energy dimensions coming our way at this time.

Living in a conscious world means that we not only listen to our body's organ/gland feelings, but learn to consciously respond to them clearly and quickly. It means expressing our Spirit's truth, rather than ignoring and suppressing that truth. Living in a conscious world is about creating sufficient safety to neutralize our defensiveness and bring our walls *down,* rather than feeling the need to build our walls *up.*

A conscious world invites our Spirit's Light of truth to reveal its Ways that fulfill our divine intent – rather than perpetuate old, defensive survival ways of the undisciplined dragon that create degeneration and self destruction (from dragon/trauma fears programmed when we had no power or choice).

I have found that the new world of the 'promised land' is not a physical place (though it certainly affects the physical world), but is rather a Way of Being centered on being true to our Spirit Self by focusing on performing the Ways of our Spirit in our lives, so our pathway goes energetically toward regeneration. This is the pathway that evolves us into the 'Golden Age of Enlightenment' we have all been waiting to experience for so long now.

****

Further information about this consciousness science is available on the internet at Dr. Allen's website: http://dgallenphd.com.

Therapists and health professionals who would like more information about who we are and how we function in the subtle energy realm of trauma memory may email me at dgallenphd@aol.com.

Author's note: See a sample of my clients' testimonials about their experiences, now available at http://DGAllenPhD.com.

About the Author

Dean G. Allen, PhD

Dr. Allen is a Wellness/Consciousness Consultant who uses an infra-red science to track and decode human symptoms and problems into organ/gland wisdom messages. When these messages are followed through proper perception and expression of each organ's function they create 'elegant solutions' to our personal challenges. Unconscious trauma memory (our history) of not being safe or able – creates a *'drag'* on our perceptions and expressions necessary to manifest our divine intent. This 'drag' can be measured and tracked by infrared science into the unconscious causes of all our human problems.

Professional experience: I have served as a Clinical Services Director for a Human Development Center; did Biofeedback Research on the Autonomic Nervous System; and worked as a Wellness and Stress Management Consultant for the Times Publishing Company and initiated the Human Enhancement Program at Innisbrook Resort in Florida. Since 1987 I have focused all my professional work on doing infrared clinical research with thousands of clients. See more at http://DGAllenPhD.com.

Education: I hold a Ph.D. in Clinical Psychology from Utah State University (1982), where I began my career doing my doctoral dissertation research using biofeedback to monitor my research on "Autonomic Nervous System Control as a Function of Imagery."

Teaching and Research Experience: I taught "The Psychology of Consciousness" from 1976 to 1981, while working at Boise State University at the Counseling Center doing my doctoral dissertation research on how *imagery ability* scientifically relates to our ability to control our autonomic nervous system using biofeedback.

From 1982 to 1987: I began the Health Enhancement Institute at Innisbrook Resort in Florida, where I taught stress management and did biofeedback with clients as a way of providing personal insights to promote personal health through personal consciousness.

In 1987 I met Joseph R. Scogna, Jr. and began using infrared science to observe how electrical energy flow patterns (from trauma memory) create dysfunctional energy-motion (e-motional dysfunction). After Joe's death in 1989, his old Apple IIE computer system became obsolete and Joe's original programmers told me the apple software they created for Joe *"could not upgraded,"* I was thus forced to create a personal computer (PC) infrared system I call "The BodyTalker." This system also uses infrared data plus our organ/gland language/functions to help decode dysfunctional energy flow patterns from unconscious trauma memory that creates our problems. [See "What is The BodyTalker" at http://DGAllenPhD.com.]

I have used this infrared science to analyze thousands of clients since 1987. I am now beginning to make this very insightful science more available to those who seek truth about themselves and desire to gain more conscious insights about their personal programming (which allows them to make life decisions more clearly and quickly).

Currently, I use these infrared organ/gland insights with all my clients to reveal their personal programming and enable them to benefit from clearer thinking to perceive and express more effectively and engage in more regenerative and productive mental, emotional and physical functioning.